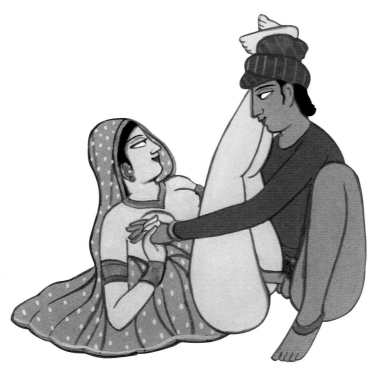

THE NEW
KAMA SUTRA

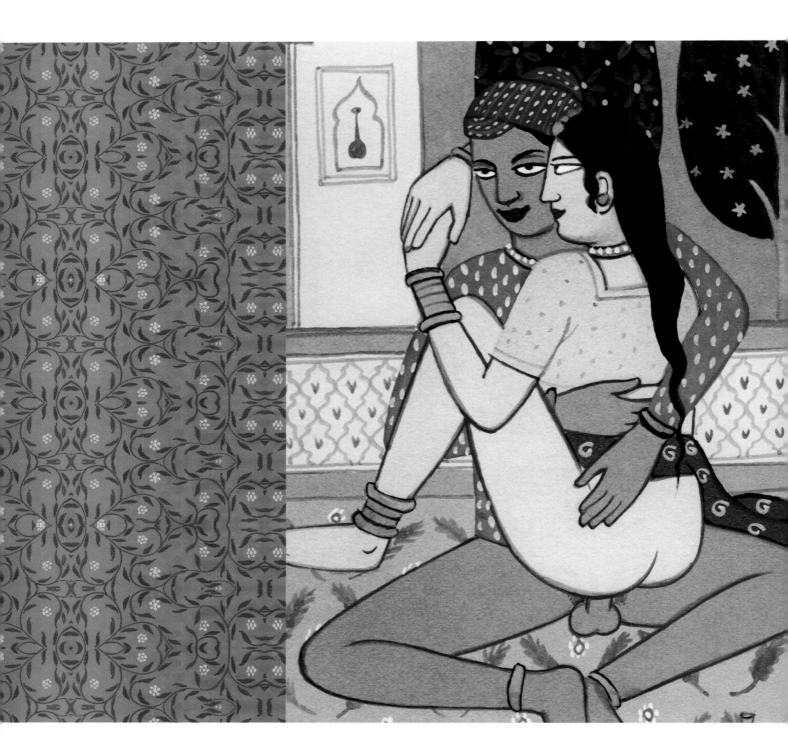

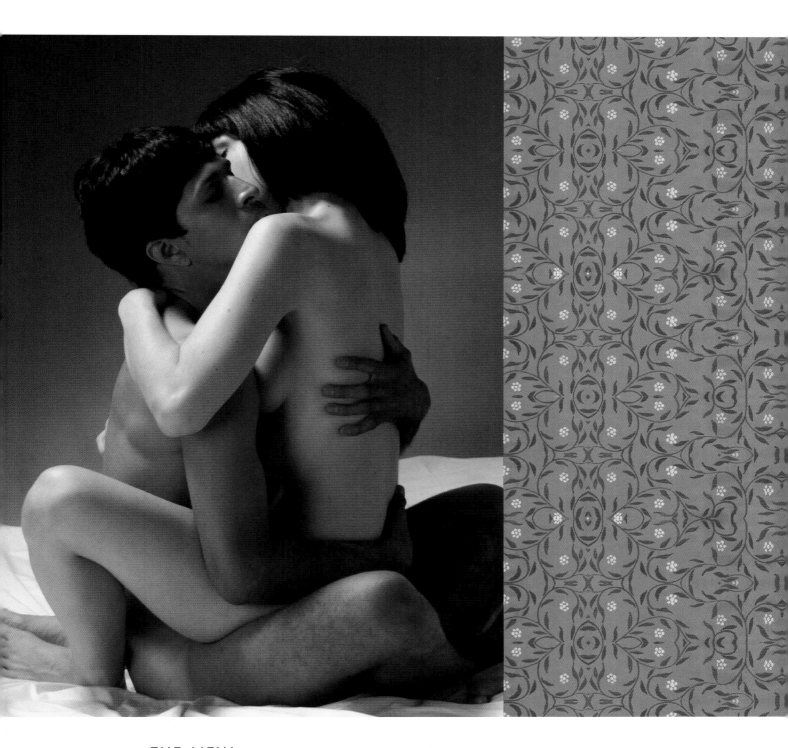

THE NEW
KAMA SUTRA

Randi Foxx

HYLAS PUBLISHING

HYLAS
PUBLISHING

Hylas Publishing®
129 Main Street, Ste. C
Irvington, NY 10533
www.hylaspublishing.com

Hylas Publishing
Publisher: Sean Moore
Publishing Director: Karen Prince
Art Director: Gus Yoo
Editorial Director: Gail Greiner
Production Manager: Wayne Ellis
Designers: Erika Lubowicki, La Tricia Watford
Editors: Marisa Iallonardo, Ward Calhoun
Assistant Editor: Mary Kate Aveni
Proofreader: Franchesca Ho Sang
Photographer: Robert Wright
Illustrations: Cybermedia

ISBN: 1-59258-184-6
ISBN13/EAN: 978-1592-58184-9

Library of Congress Cataloging-in-Publication Data available upon request.
Printed and bound in Singapore

First American Edition published in 2006
10 9 8 7 6 5 4 3 2 1

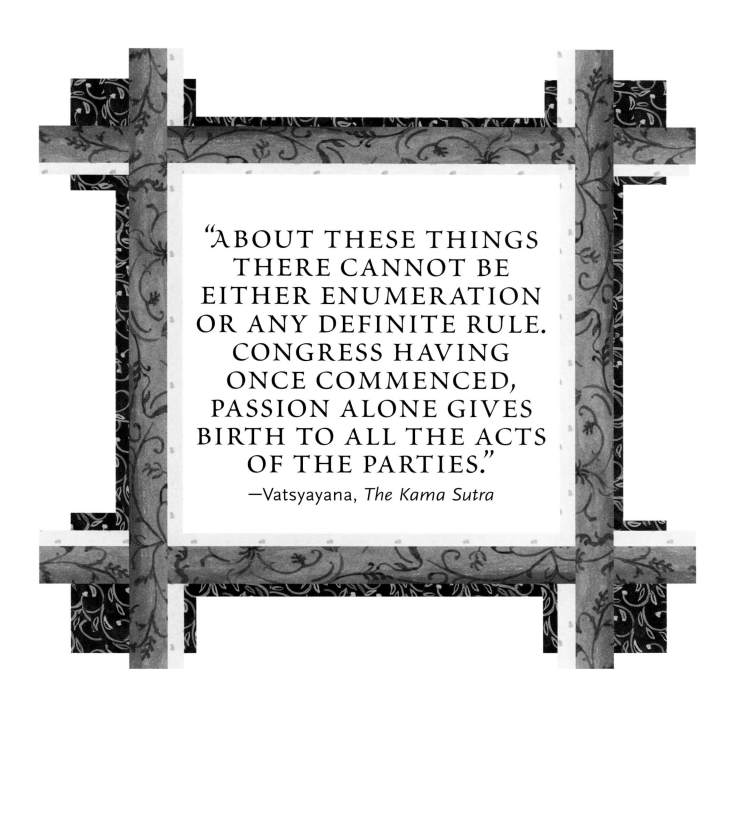

"ABOUT THESE THINGS
THERE CANNOT BE
EITHER ENUMERATION
OR ANY DEFINITE RULE.
CONGRESS HAVING
ONCE COMMENCED,
PASSION ALONE GIVES
BIRTH TO ALL THE ACTS
OF THE PARTIES."

—Vatsyayana, *The Kama Sutra*

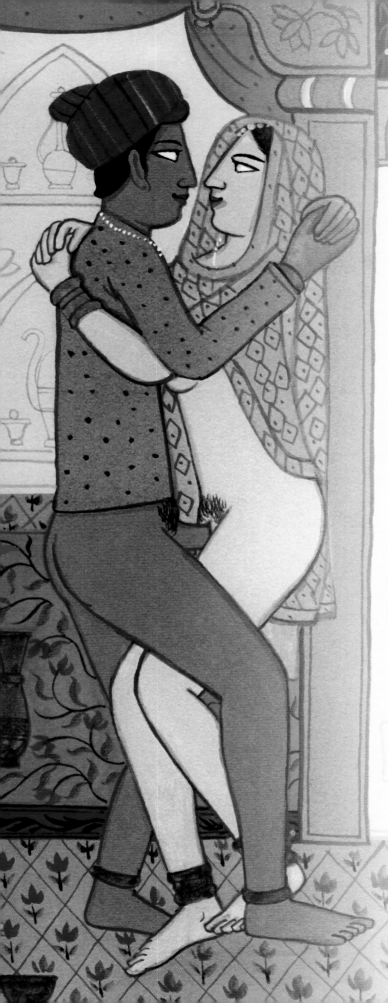

CONTENTS

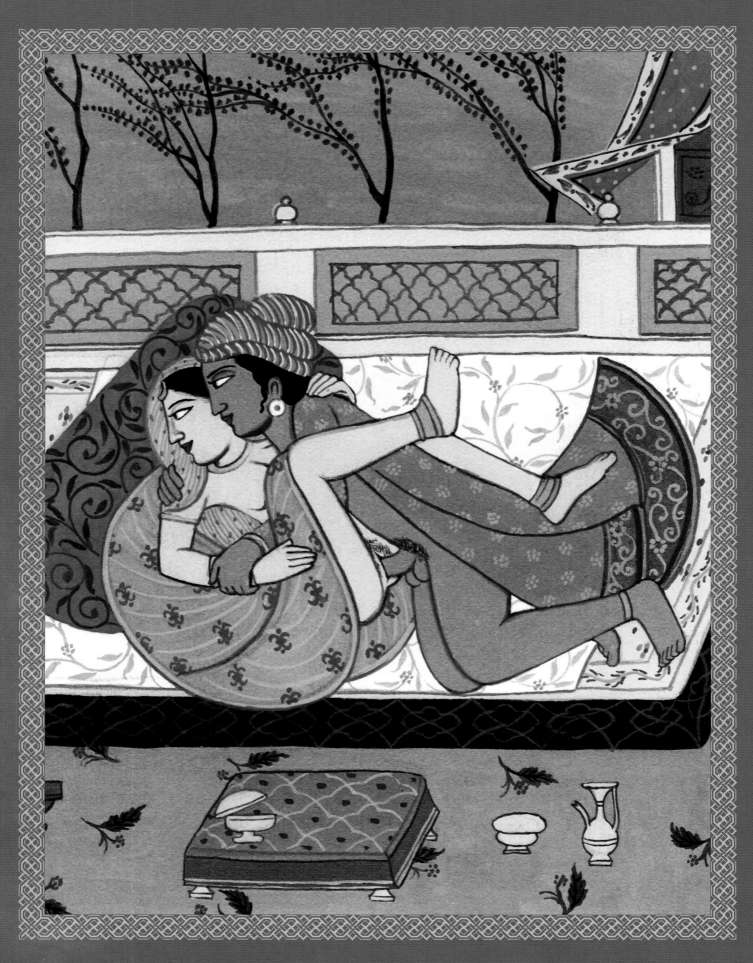

INTRODUCTION

The *Kama Sutra* is shrouded in mystery. Who wrote it? When? Is it really an ancient guide to sex? These questions have raised many misconceptions about the infamous text. The *Kama Sutra* is, in fact, an ancient guide to sex. But, rather than merely a list of positions, the original *Kama Sutra* is a treatise on love, filled with hundreds of scenarios, words of advice, and suggestions on everything from how to touch a woman—"... the man should rub the yoni of the woman with his hand and fingers... "—to how to react to a woman's anger—"... the lover should attempt to reconcile her with conciliatory words ...". Written for men, the original *Kama Sutra* is widely considered to be the definitive work on love in Sanskrit literature.

Translated to mean "Aphorisms on Love," the *Kama Sutra*, also known as the Kamasutram, was believed to have been written by Vatsyayana, a scholar in medieval India, who was thought to have lived between the 1st and 6th centuries. The *Kama Sutra* is sometimes confused with another popular Indian text on love, *The Ananga-Ranga*, which focused on the love between husband and wife—possibly written in the mid 12th century. The *Ananga-Ranga* also described various positions and techniques for keeping love strong and sexual discovery important. Many of the positions thought to be from the *Kama Sutra* are actually from the *Ananga-Ranga*. Indeed, approximately one quarter of the positions in these pages are based on that text.

The *Kama Sutra*, which is the main focus of this book, is broken down into 35 chapters, each on a central theme important to Indian men of the day. These chapters cover everything from the importance of love, to the "means of attracting others to oneself," to courtship and marriage. As interesting as it is to read advice on dealing with the women of the harem or about how to decide which wife to shower with the most attention, this aspect of the text is valued mainly as a historical document. While only about 20 percent of the *Kama Sutra* is dedicated to sexual positions, including foreplay, oral sex, and orgasms, it is that 20 percent that is the legacy of the *Kama Sutra*.

Many books have been written about the positions in the *Kama Sutra* and the *Ananga-Ranga*, mostly illustrated with elaborate Indian paintings. While these illustrations are without a doubt beautiful, they leave the modern couple thinking: That's impossible! Can we do that? Did these women really put their legs behind their ears? Could the men possibly hold up their lovers and shoot birds at the same time? Perhaps they did. Perhaps they could. But the likelihood is that the average person today cannot. So, in *The New Kama Sutra*, gone are the birds, the guns, and the yoga masters. The ancient Indian positions are shown in all their beauty and detail, and then interpreted by a modern couple with a moderate flexibility range. We've taken the *Kama Sutra* positions down to their essence to show that anyone can perform these moves. On the following pages, you will discover ways to incorporate the *Kama Sutra* positions into your regular sex life: What to do if you're not as flexible as you'd like; if he's not as strong as he thinks; or if you're both just looking to break out of the routine and change things up a bit. Because, in truth, Vatsyayana understood that there are no rules in sex. He continuously stressed the idea that imagination should play a key role and love should be the most lasting pleasure of all. So, let your legs fall where they may. Move your hands in whichever direction feels good. And, most importantly, permit passion to enter, take over, and last a lifetime.

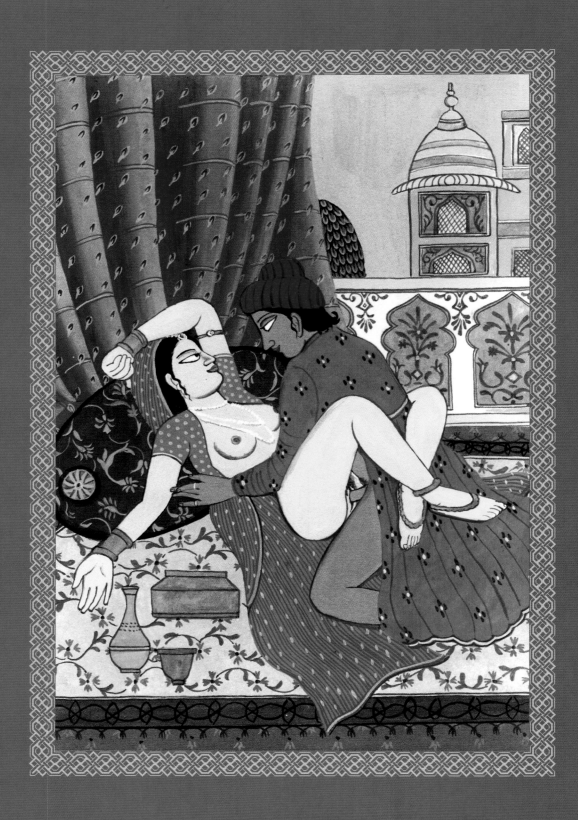

1
TWINING POSITIONS

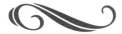

The Twining Positions are the most passionate of all the positions in the Kama Sutra. They are also one of the least complicated.

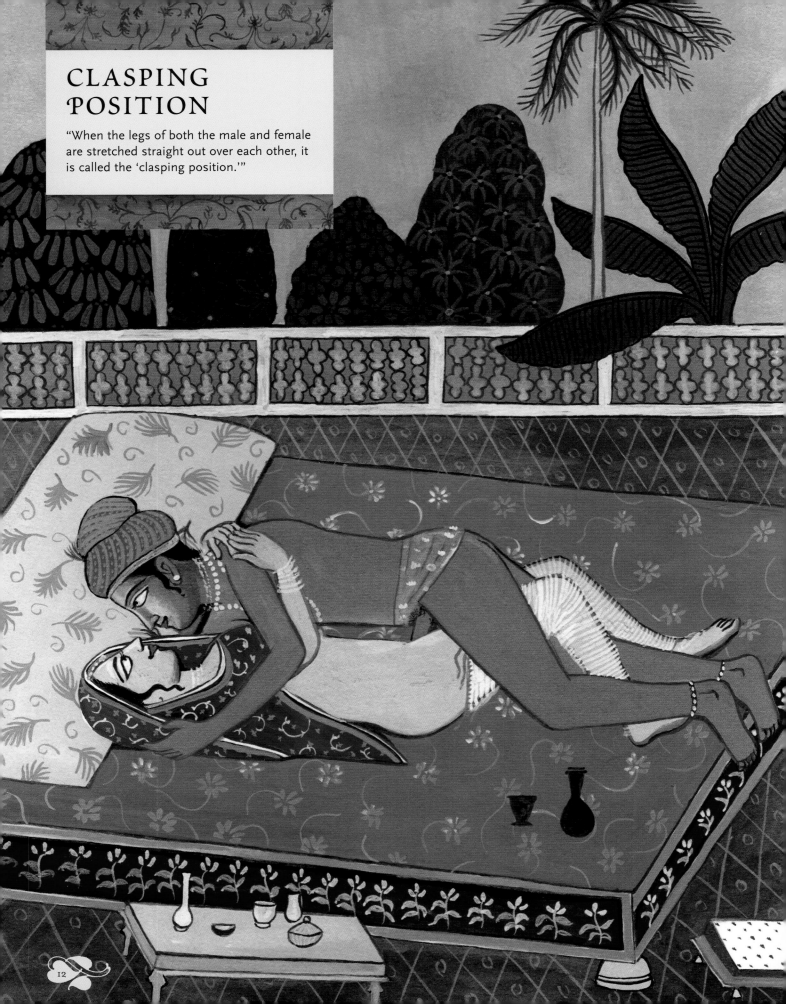

CLASPING POSITION

"When the legs of both the male and female are stretched straight out over each other, it is called the 'clasping position.'"

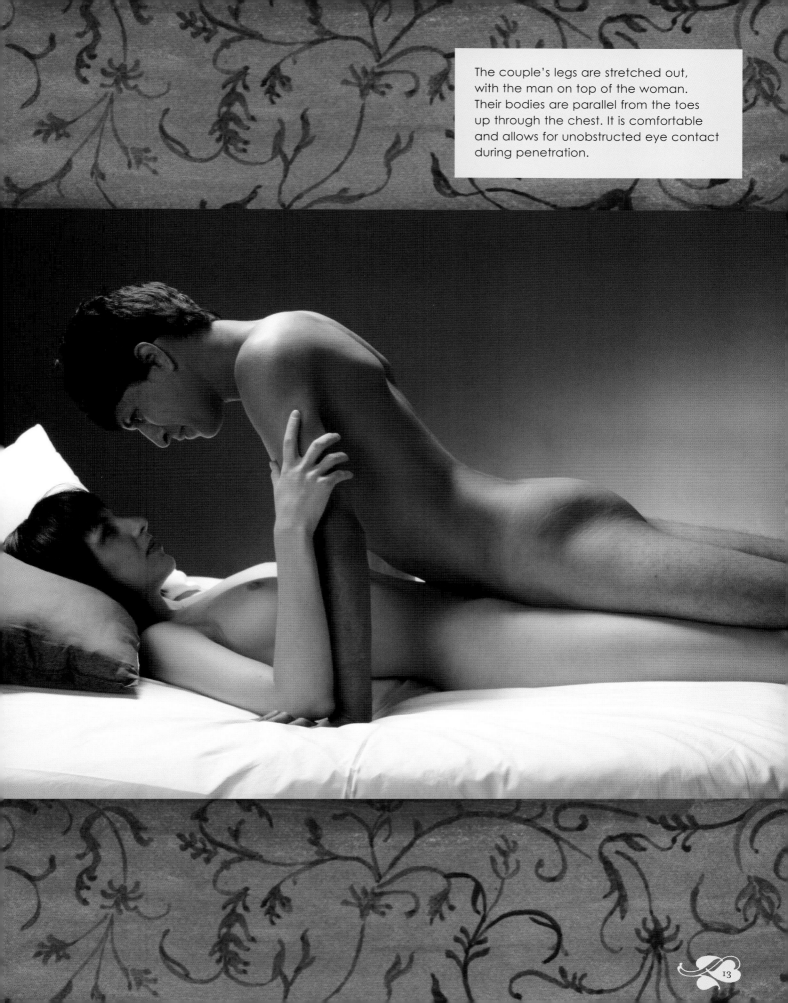

The couple's legs are stretched out, with the man on top of the woman. Their bodies are parallel from the toes up through the chest. It is comfortable and allows for unobstructed eye contact during penetration.

13

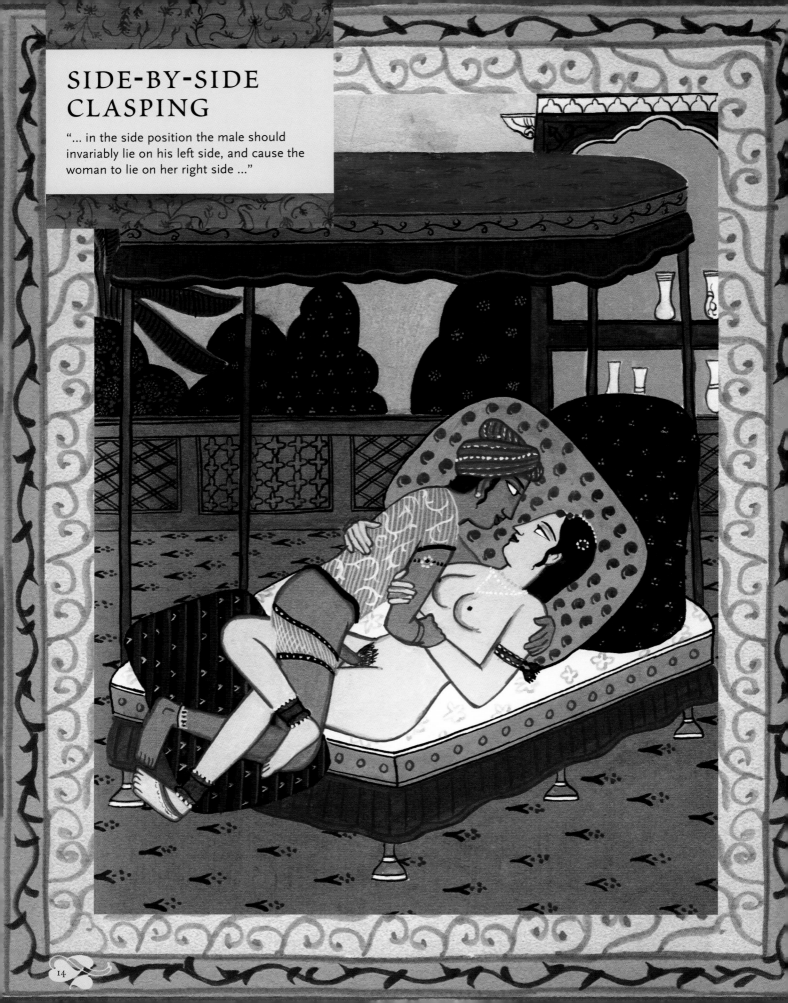

SIDE-BY-SIDE CLASPING

"... in the side position the male should invariably lie on his left side, and cause the woman to lie on her right side ..."

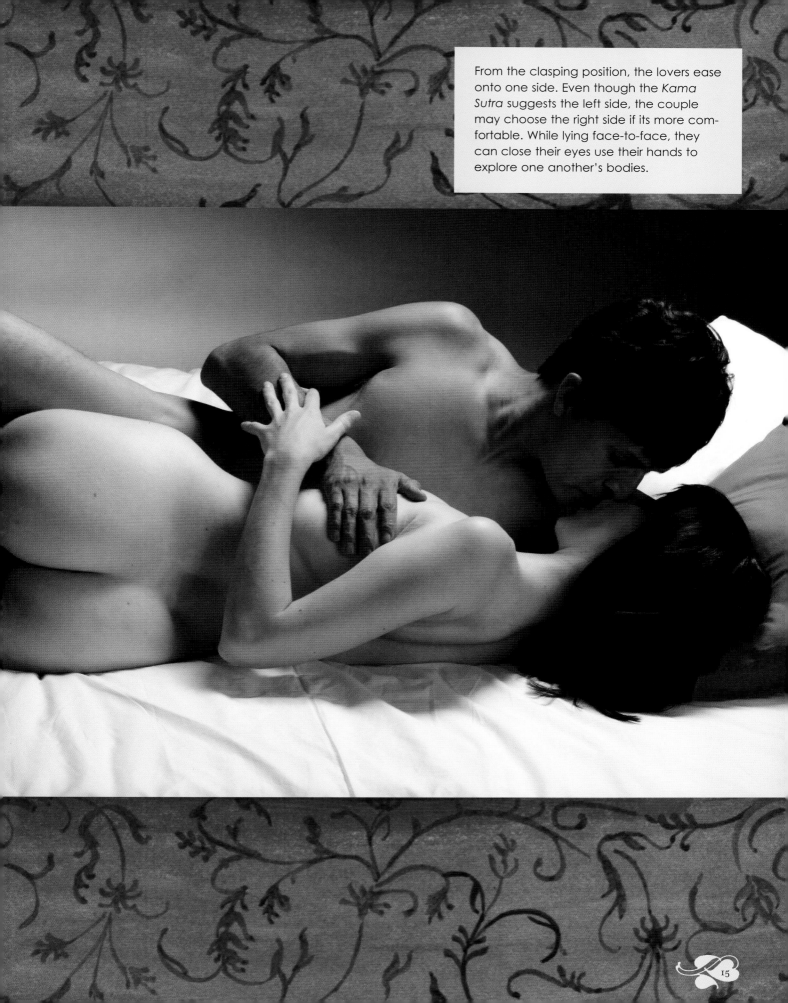

From the clasping position, the lovers ease onto one side. Even though the *Kama Sutra* suggests the left side, the couple may choose the right side if its more comfortable. While lying face-to-face, they can close their eyes use their hands to explore one another's bodies.

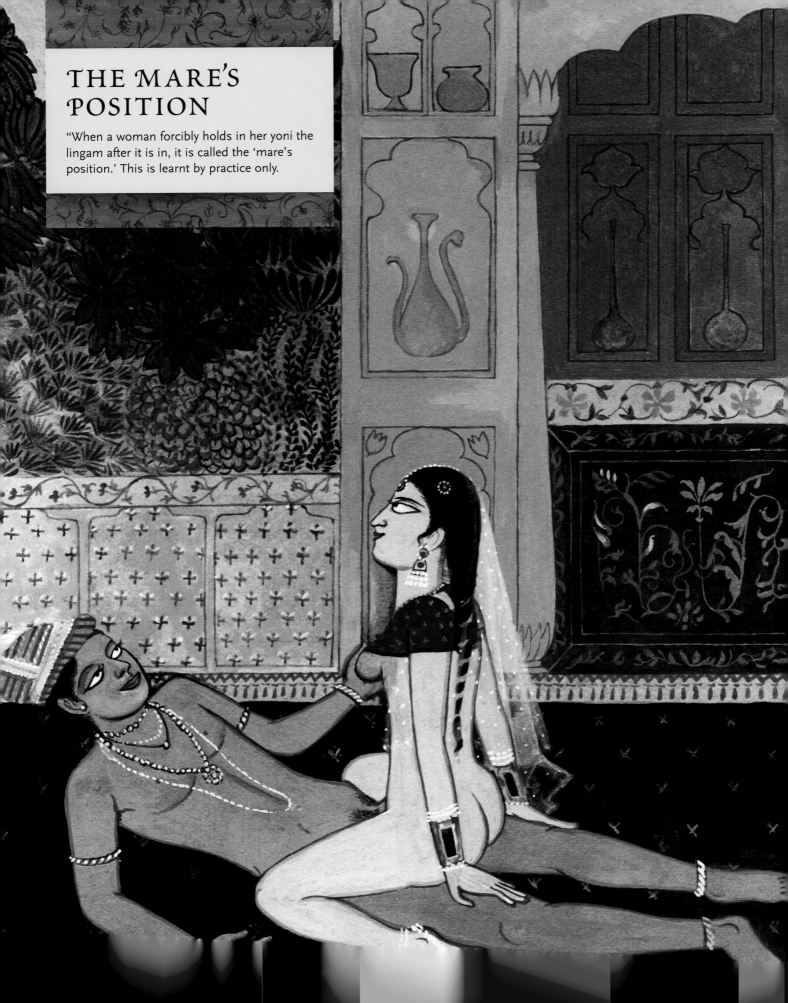

THE MARE'S POSITION

"When a woman forcibly holds in her yoni the lingam after it is in, it is called the 'mare's position.' This is learnt by practice only."

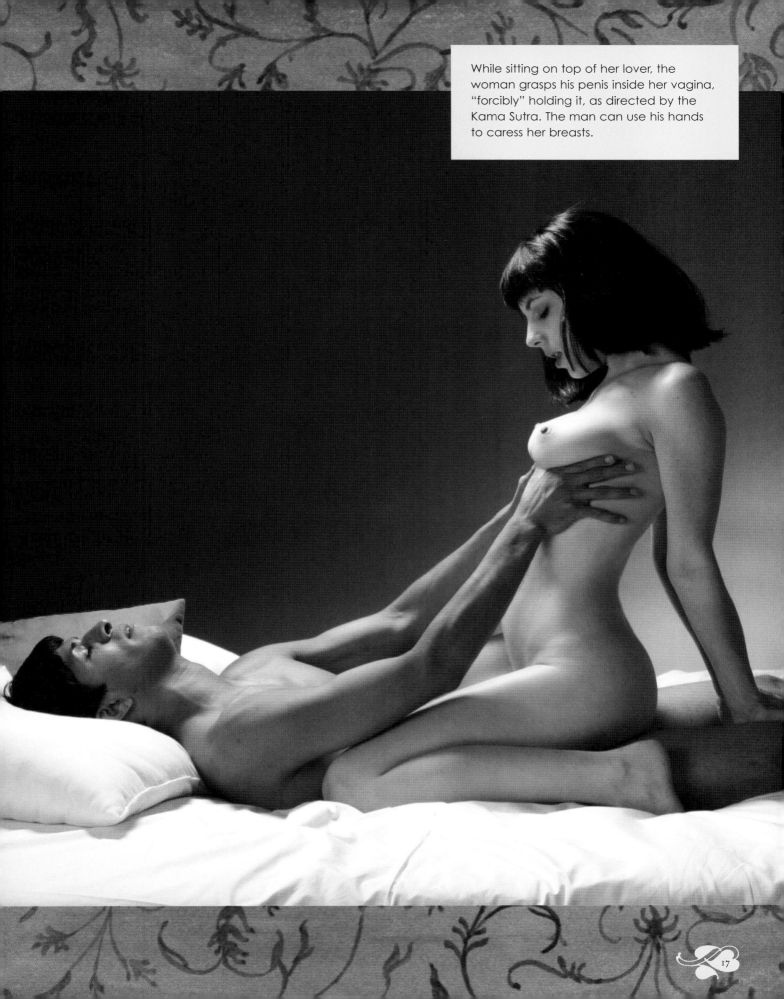

While sitting on top of her lover, the woman grasps his penis inside her vagina, "forcibly" holding it, as directed by the Kama Sutra. The man can use his hands to caress her breasts.

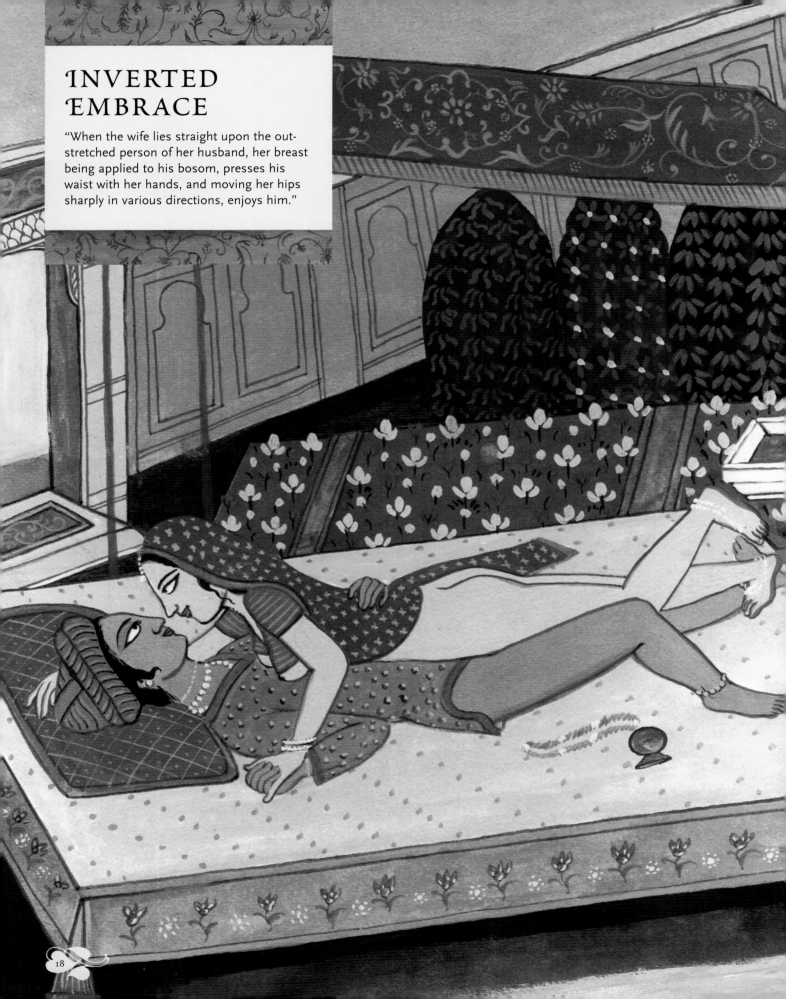

INVERTED EMBRACE

"When the wife lies straight upon the out-stretched person of her husband, her breast being applied to his bosom, presses his waist with her hands, and moving her hips sharply in various directions, enjoys him."

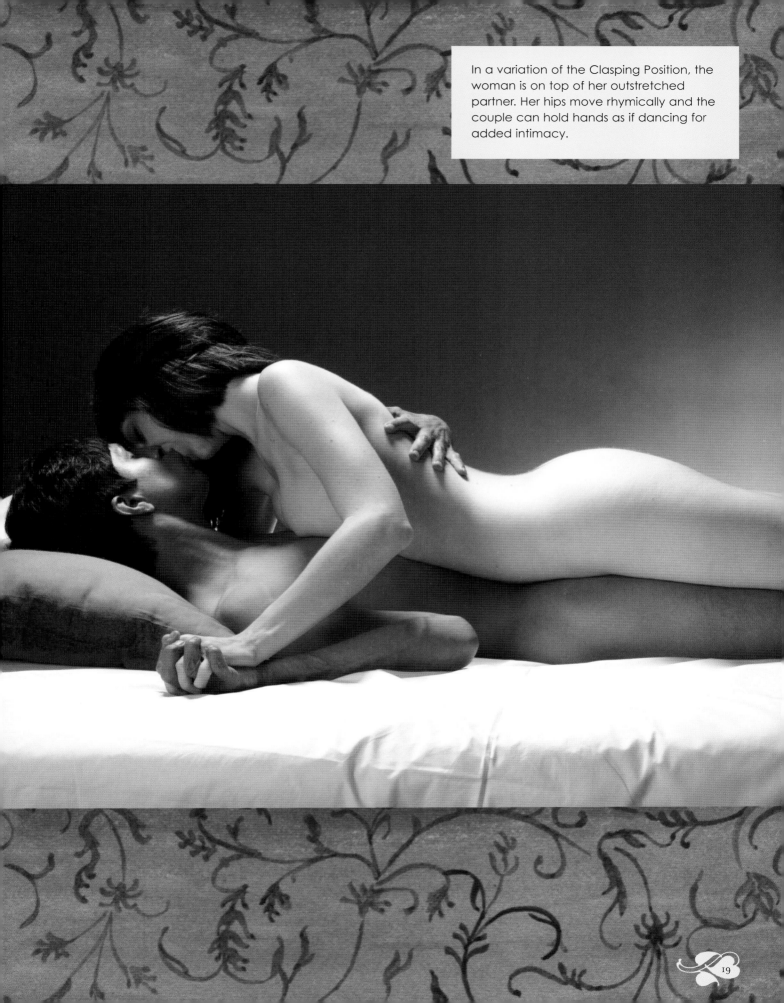

In a variation of the Clasping Position, the woman is on top of her outstretched partner. Her hips move rhymically and the couple can hold hands as if dancing for added intimacy.

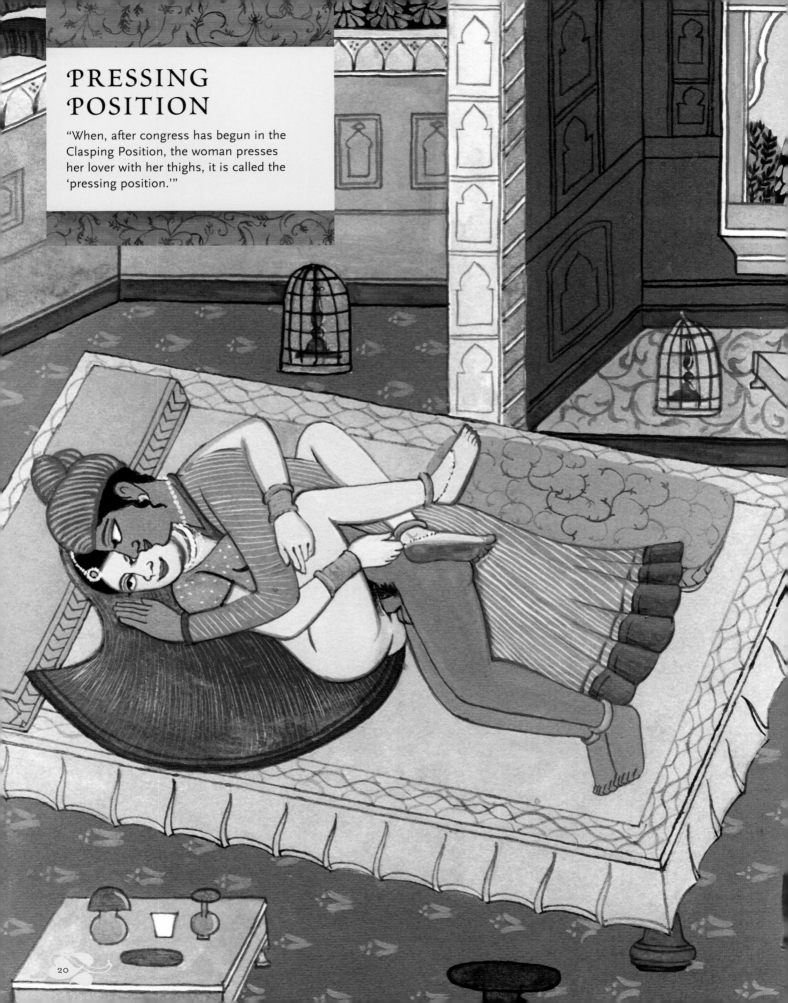

PRESSING
POSITION

"When, after congress has begun in the Clasping Position, the woman presses her lover with her thighs, it is called the 'pressing position.'"

The man is on top of the woman, as she wraps her legs around him as if scaling a tree. She can either cross her legs over his back or hold them up in the air if it is not too difficult.

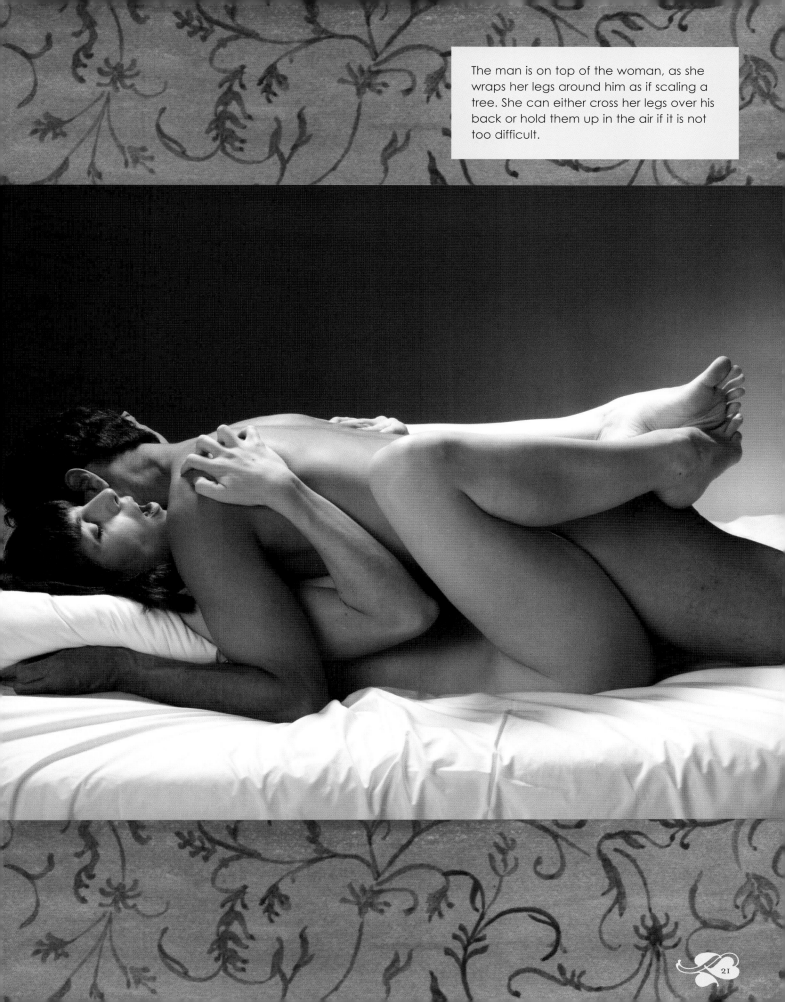

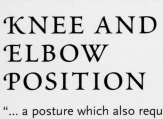

KNEE AND ELBOW POSITION

"... a posture which also requires great bodily strength in the man. Both stand opposite to each other, and the husband passes his two arms under his wife's knees, supporting her upon the inner elbows; he then raises her as high as his waist, and enjoys her, whilst she must clasp his neck with both her hands."

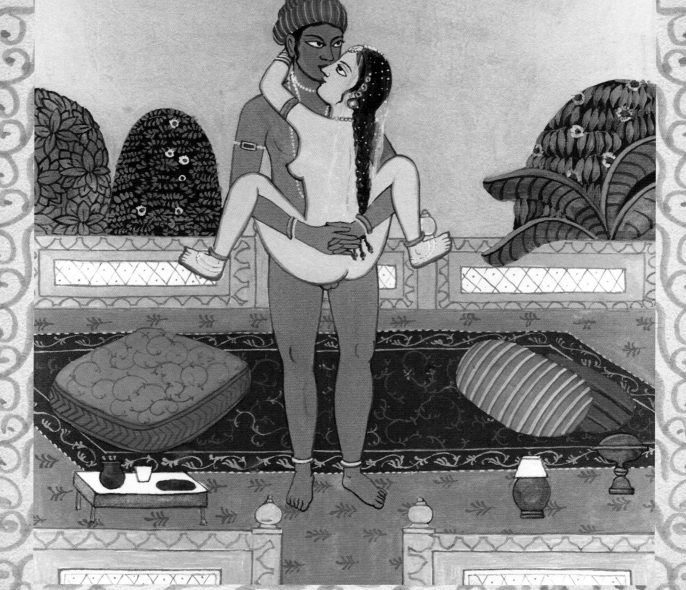

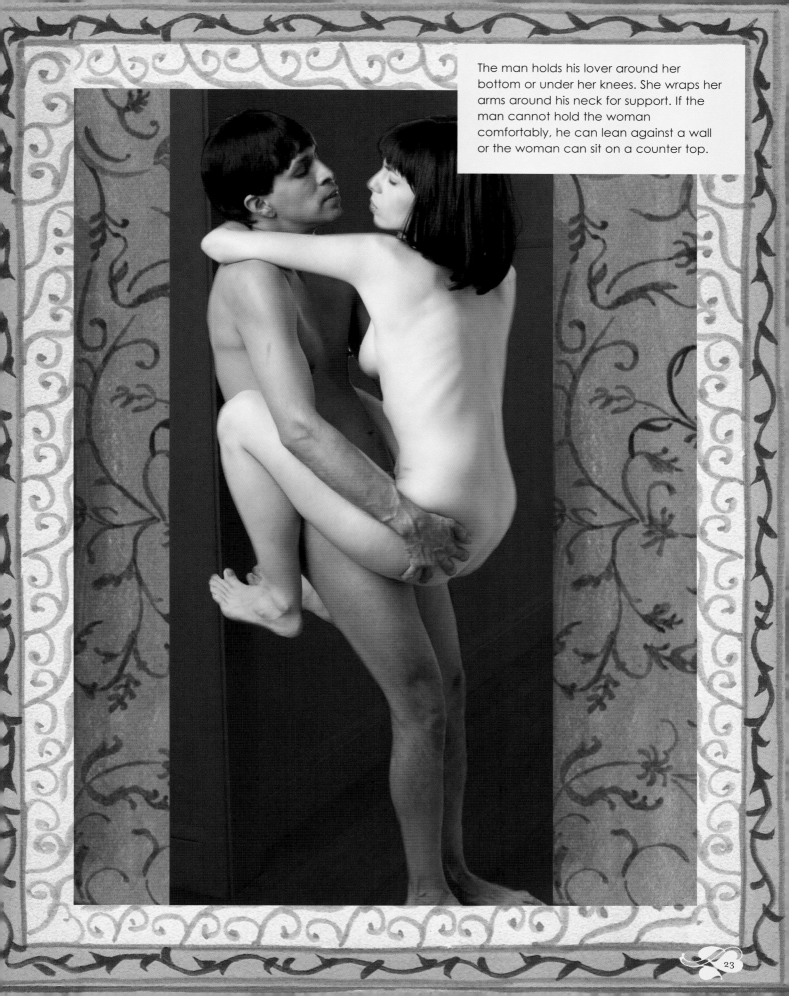

The man holds his lover around her bottom or under her knees. She wraps her arms around his neck for support. If the man cannot hold the woman comfortably, he can lean against a wall or the woman can sit on a counter top.

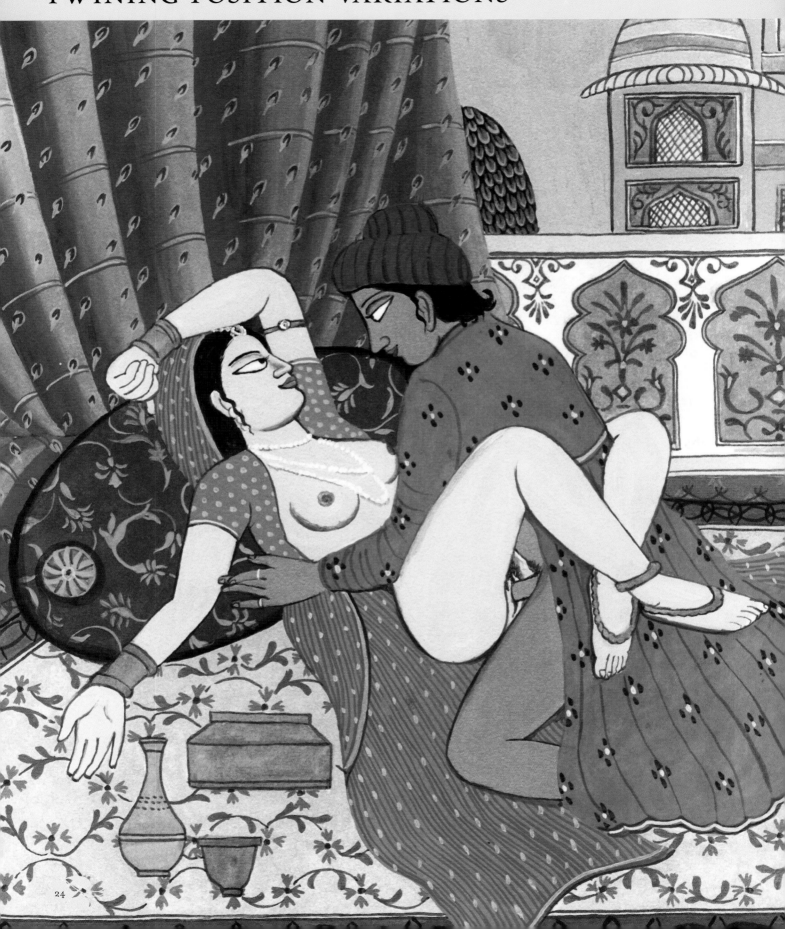

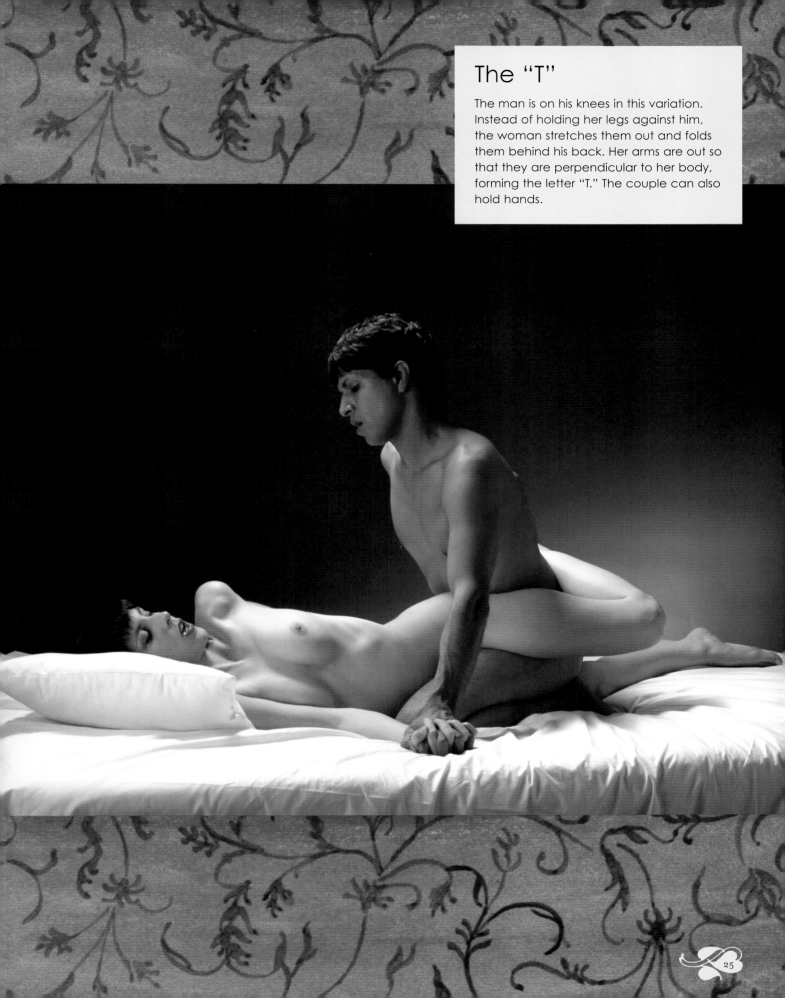

The "T"

The man is on his knees in this variation. Instead of holding her legs against him, the woman stretches them out and folds them behind his back. Her arms are out so that they are perpendicular to her body, forming the letter "T." The couple can also hold hands.

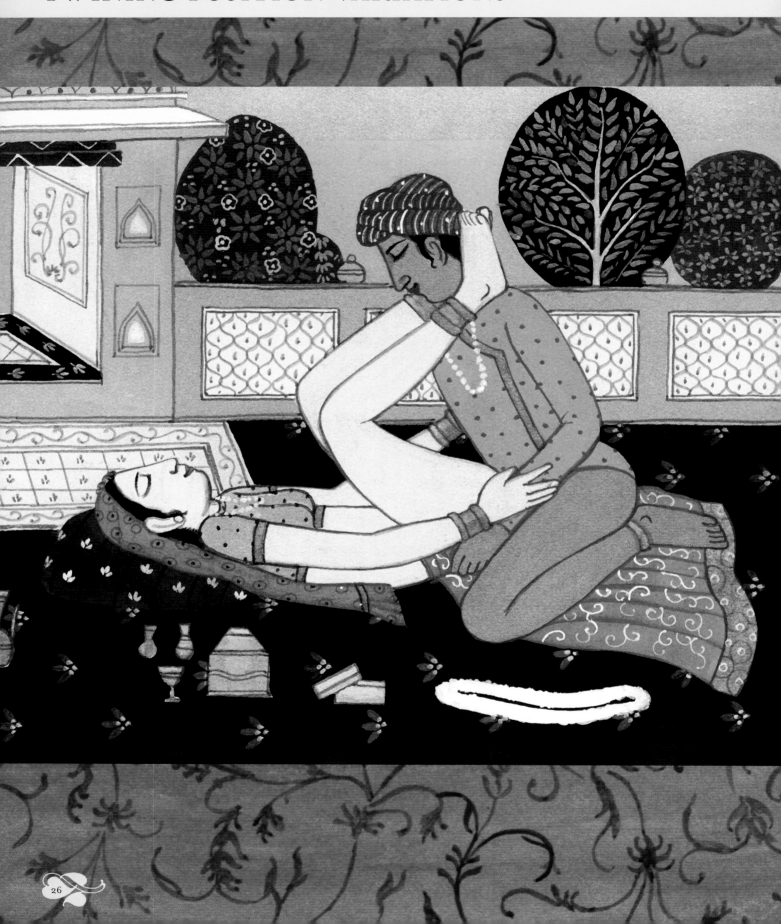

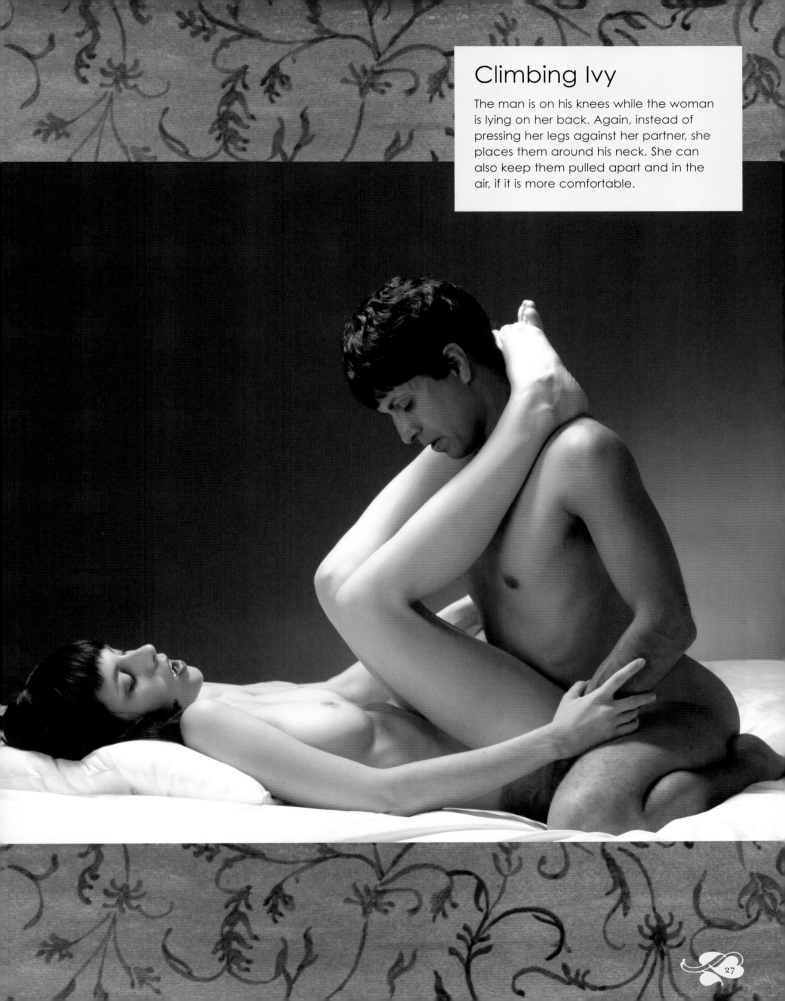

Climbing Ivy

The man is on his knees while the woman is lying on her back. Again, instead of pressing her legs against her partner, she places them around his neck. She can also keep them pulled apart and in the air, if it is more comfortable.

27

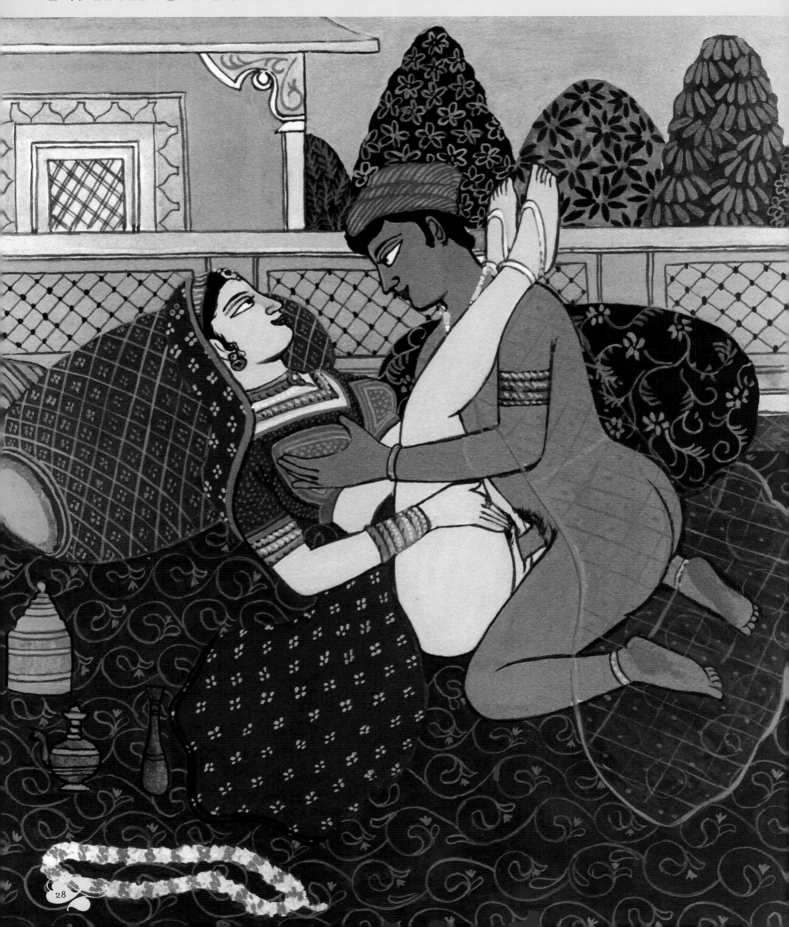

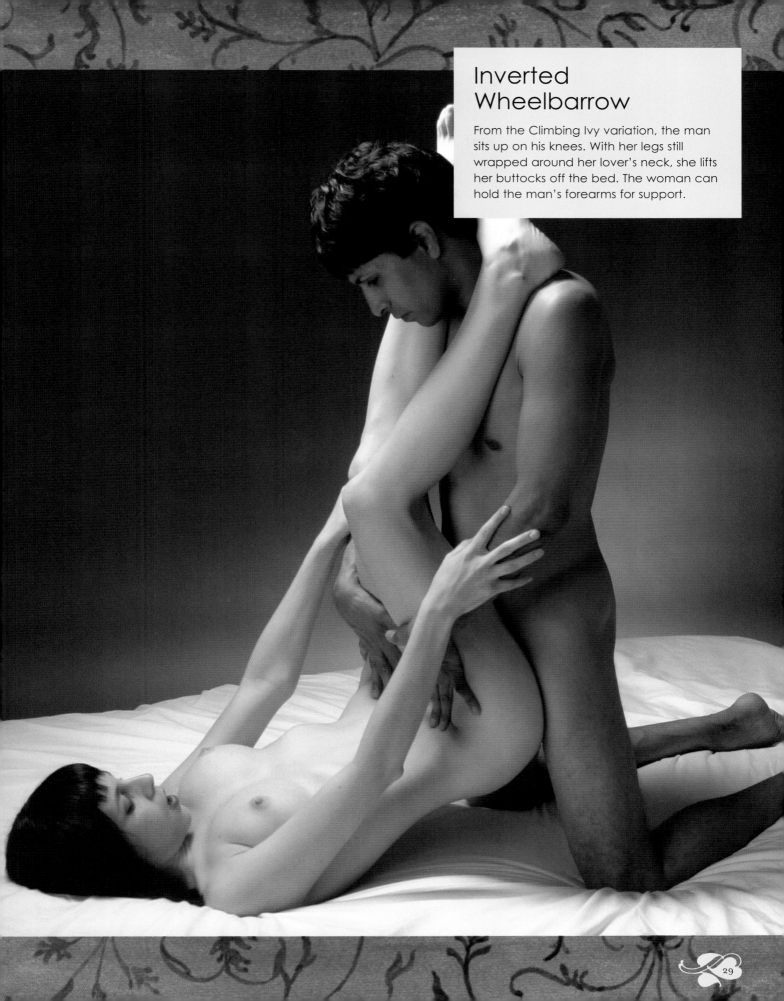

Inverted Wheelbarrow

From the Climbing Ivy variation, the man sits up on his knees. With her legs still wrapped around her lover's neck, she lifts her buttocks off the bed. The woman can hold the man's forearms for support.

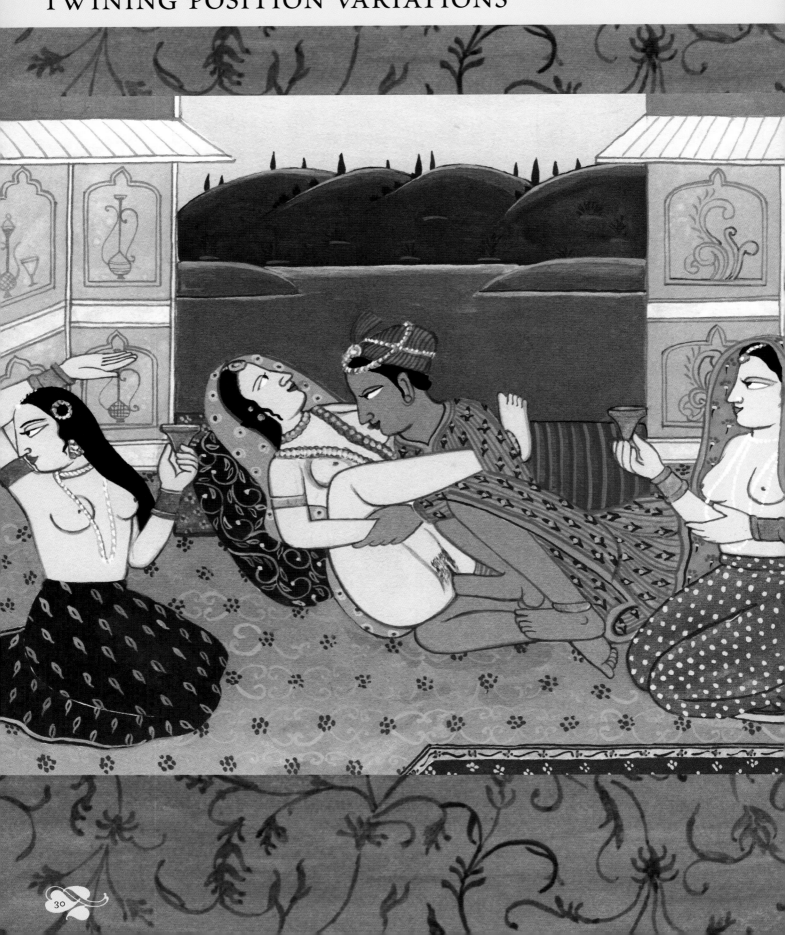

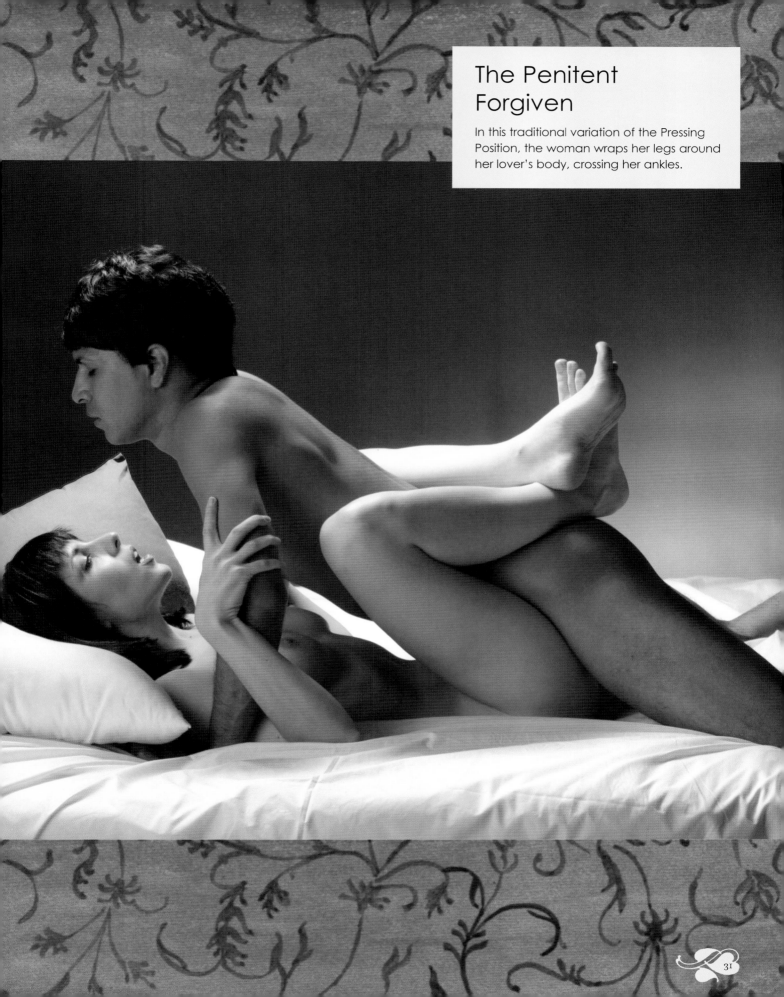

The Penitent Forgiven

In this traditional variation of the Pressing Position, the woman wraps her legs around her lover's body, crossing her ankles.

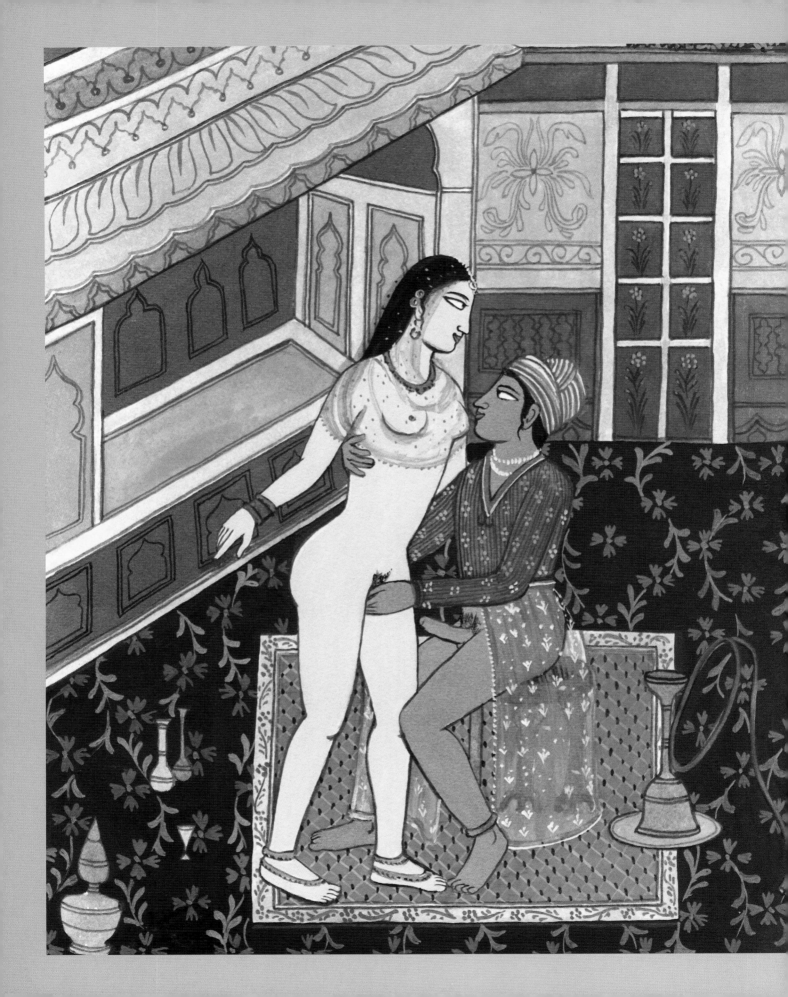

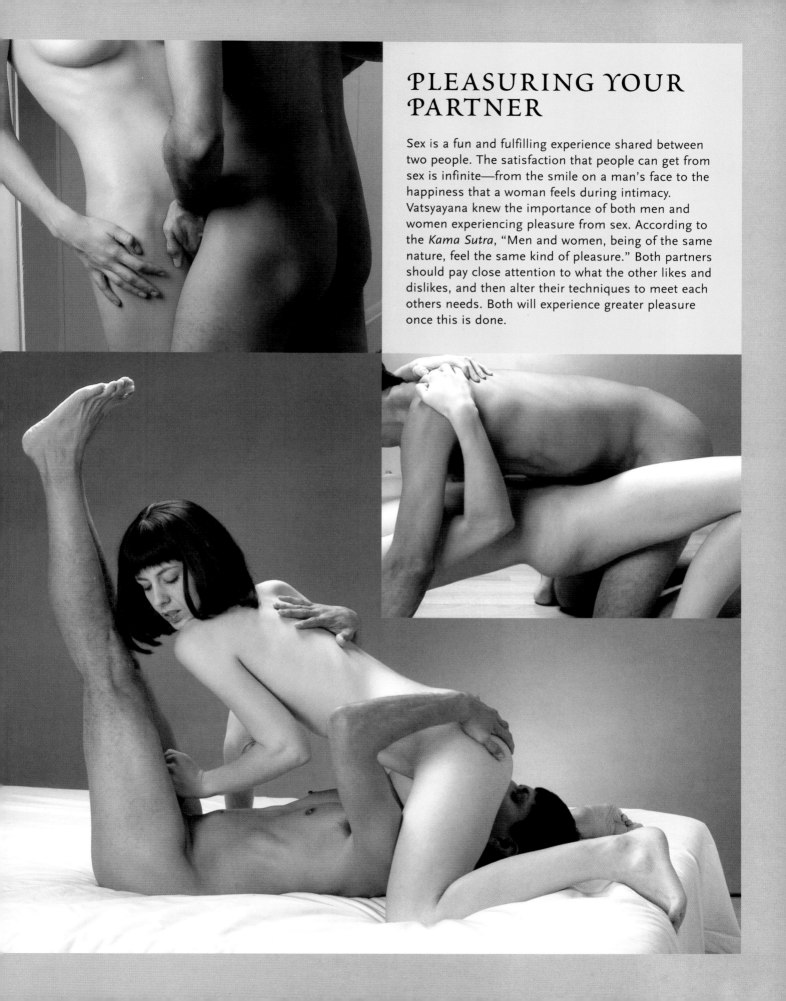

PLEASURING YOUR PARTNER

Sex is a fun and fulfilling experience shared between two people. The satisfaction that people can get from sex is infinite—from the smile on a man's face to the happiness that a woman feels during intimacy. Vatsyayana knew the importance of both men and women experiencing pleasure from sex. According to the *Kama Sutra*, "Men and women, being of the same nature, feel the same kind of pleasure." Both partners should pay close attention to what the other likes and dislikes, and then alter their techniques to meet each others needs. Both will experience greater pleasure once this is done.

The *Kama Sutra* also spends several chapters focusing on the pleasure of the woman. It states, "... while a man is doing to the woman what he likes best during congress, he should always make a point of pressing those parts of the body on which she turns her eyes." Intense pleasure is achieved not only by receiving, but by giving. There is nothing more satisfying or stimulating than making your partner happy, or experiencing new things together. This is the basis of Vatsyayana's sex theory.

Vatsyayana encouraged touching. Gently touching her body before, during, and after sex will make her respond in wonderful ways. Understanding where the man likes to be touched, will cause him to have the same pleasurable experience. These small actions make the couple feel more intimate, and will prepare their bodies for the pleasure to come.

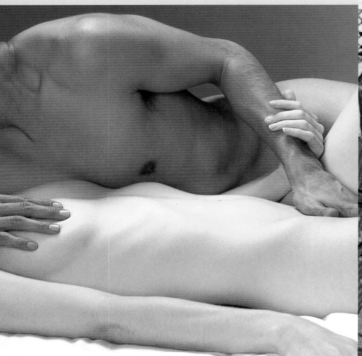

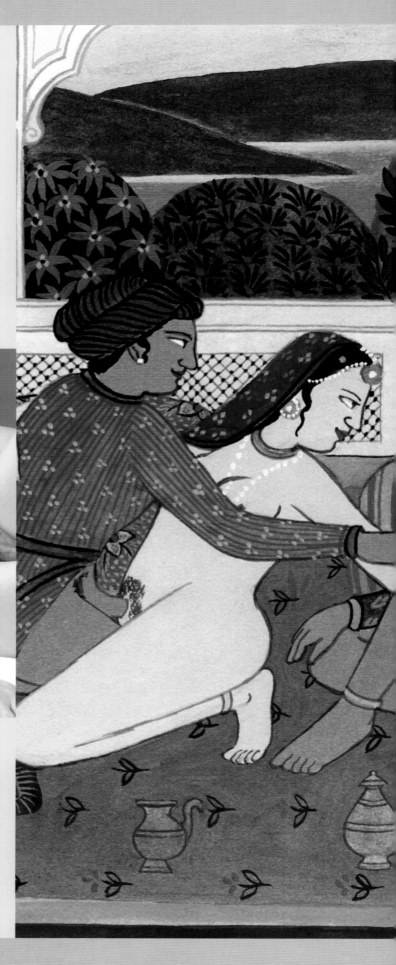

"INTENSE PLEASURE IS ATTAINED NOT ONLY BY RECEIVING, BUT BY GIVING."

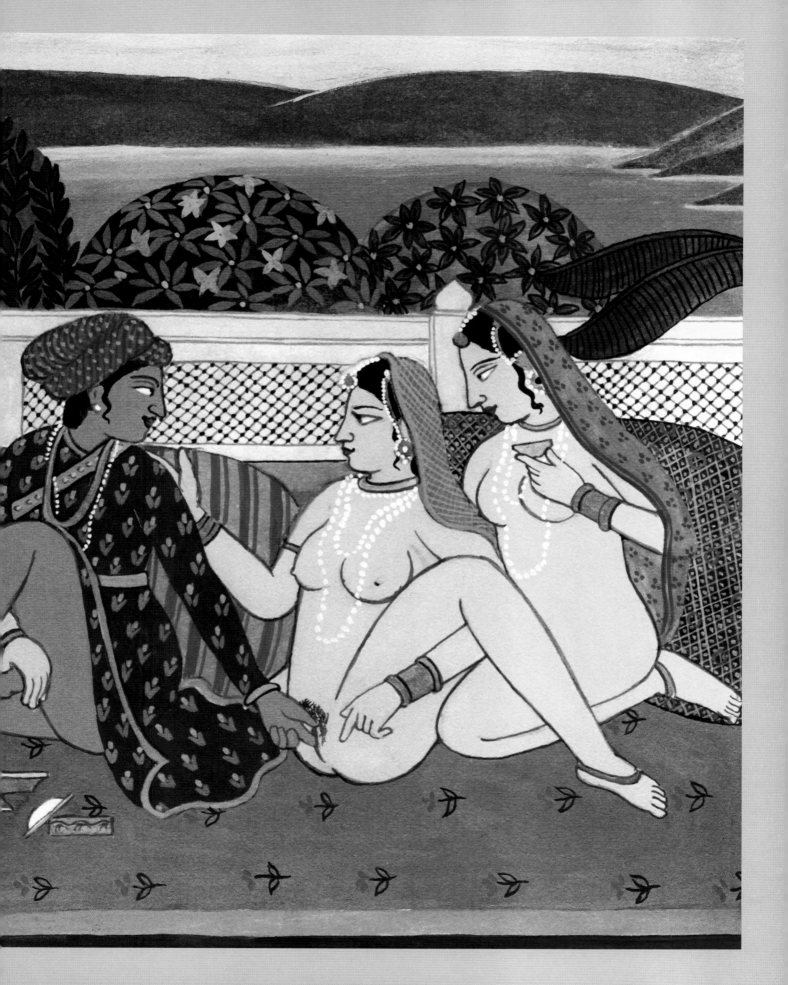

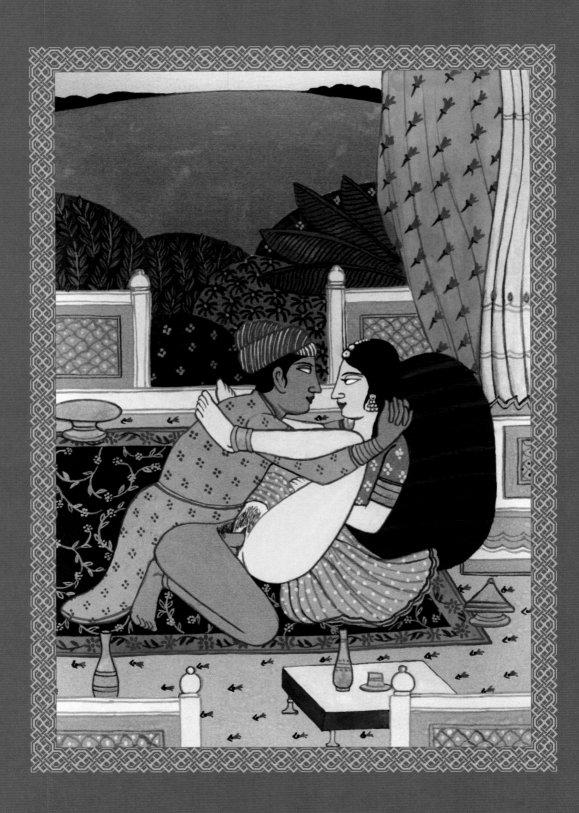

OPEN
POSITIONS

2

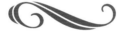

Keeping the vagina wide open is the basis of the Open Positions. They are especially comfortable for a couple where the man's penis is large compared to the woman's vagina. They allow for deep penetration and eye contact. Done face-to-face Open Positions encourage both intimacy and trust.

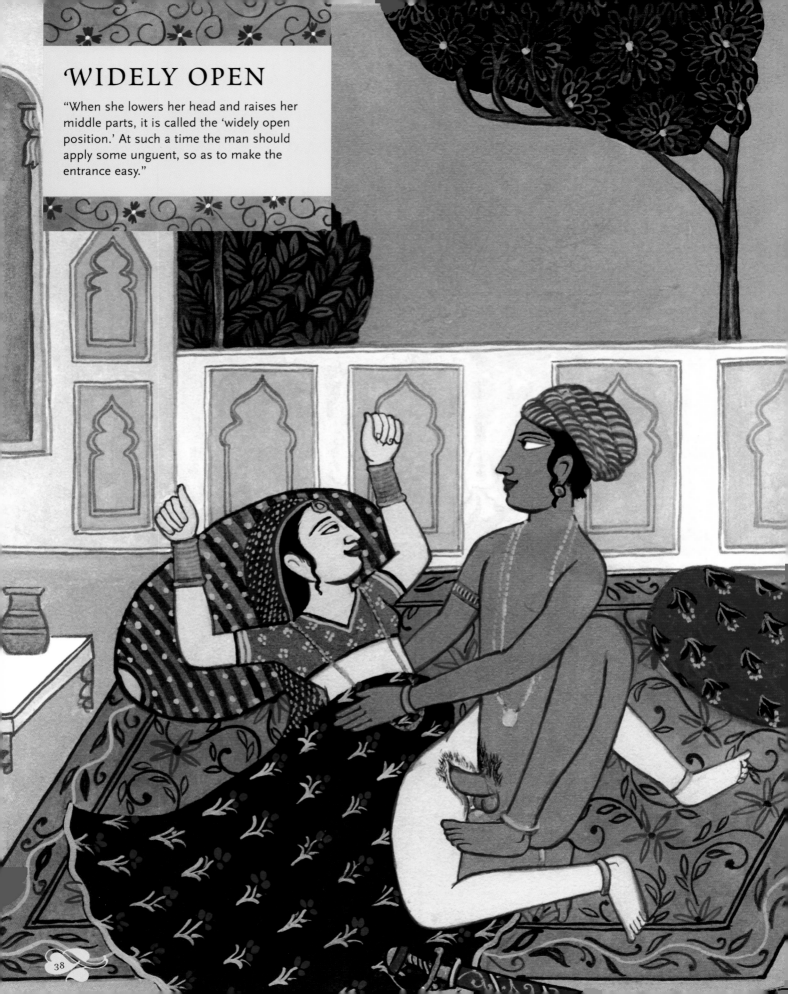

WIDELY OPEN

"When she lowers her head and raises her middle parts, it is called the 'widely open position.' At such a time the man should apply some unguent, so as to make the entrance easy."

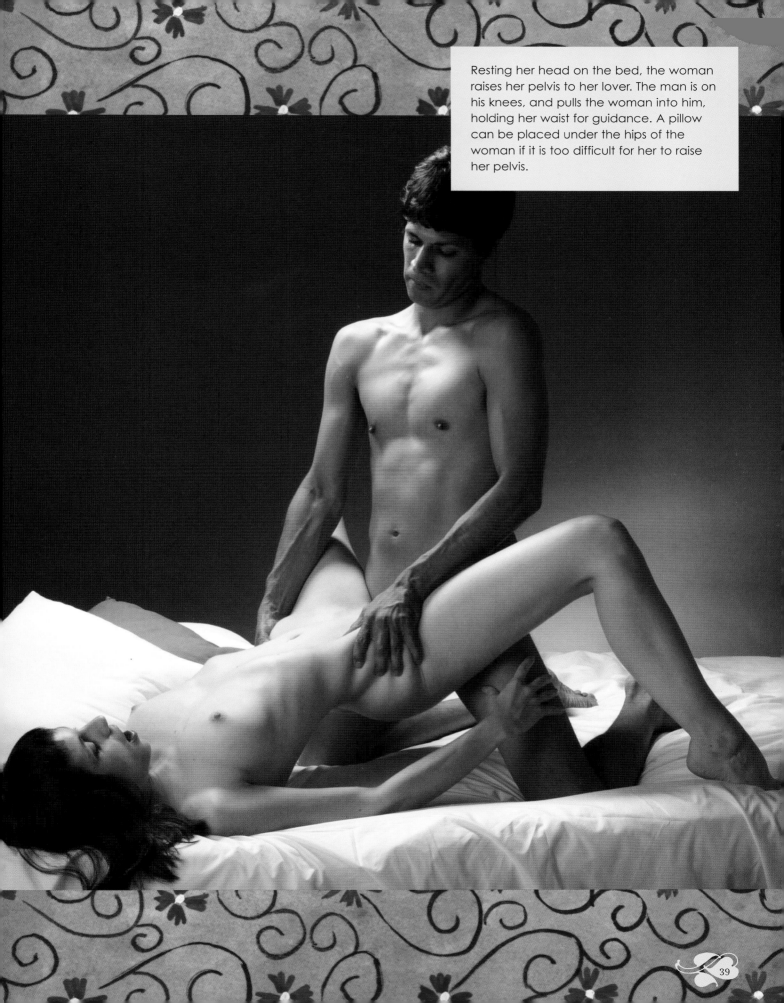

Resting her head on the bed, the woman raises her pelvis to her lover. The man is on his knees, and pulls the woman into him, holding her waist for guidance. A pillow can be placed under the hips of the woman if it is too difficult for her to raise her pelvis.

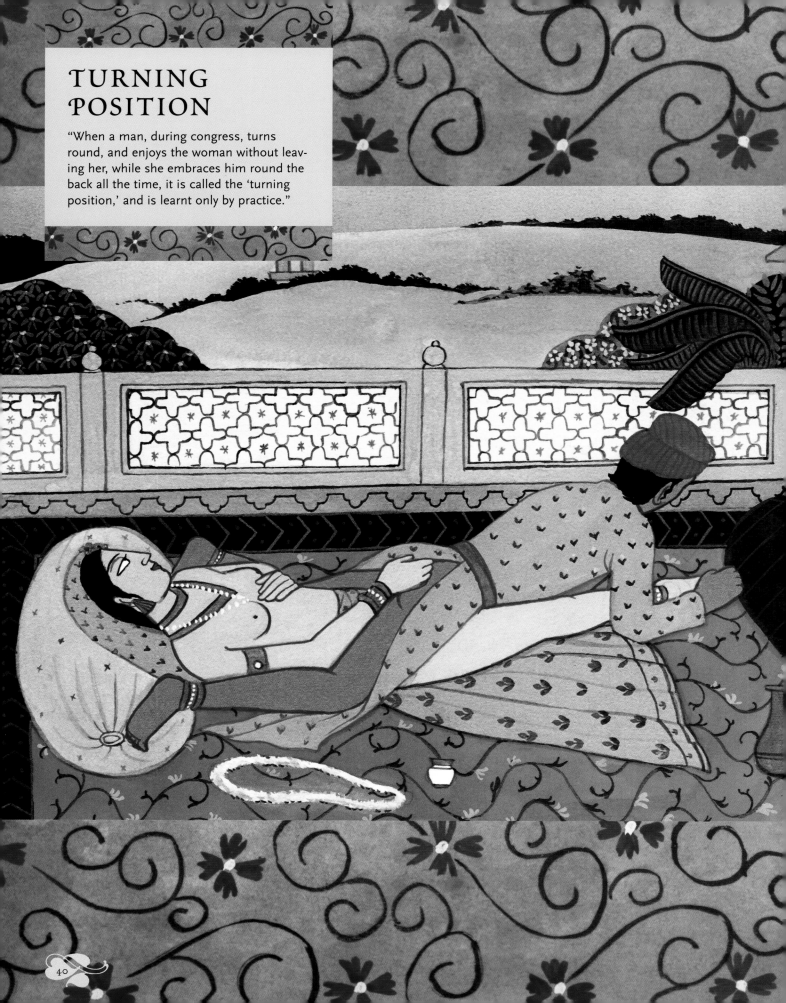

TURNING POSITION

"When a man, during congress, turns round, and enjoys the woman without leaving her, while she embraces him round the back all the time, it is called the 'turning position,' and is learnt only by practice."

The woman lies on her back and the man enters her. Without leaving his lover, he slowly turns his body around until it forms a complete circle. As stated in the Kama Sutra, it may take a bit of practice to master this difficult position.

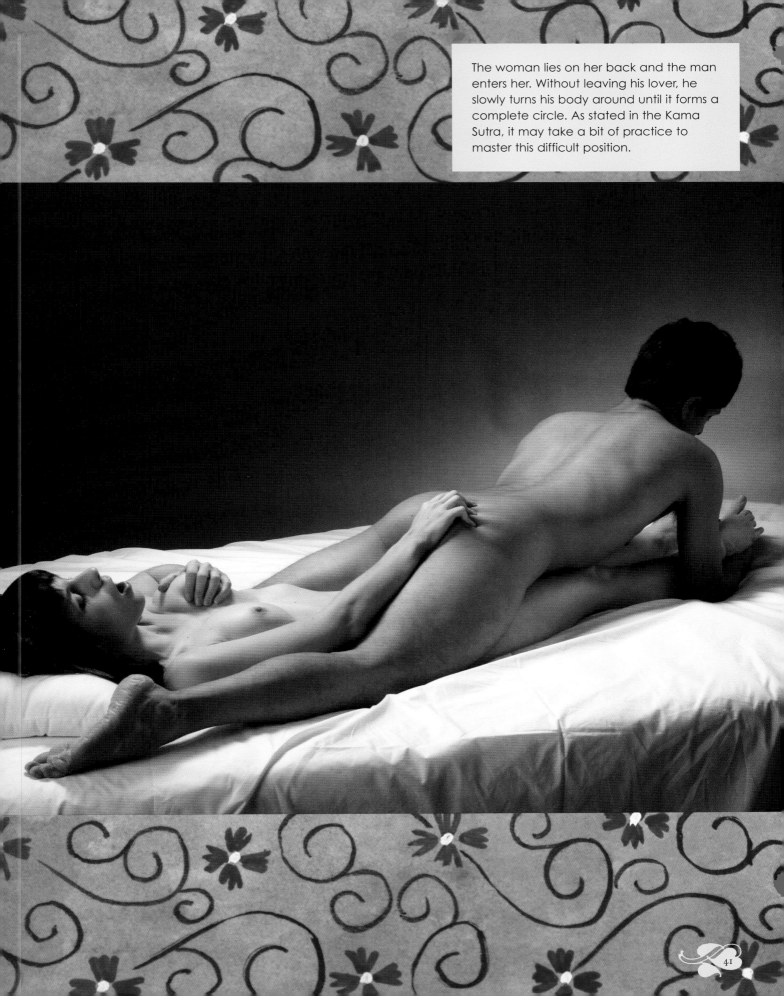

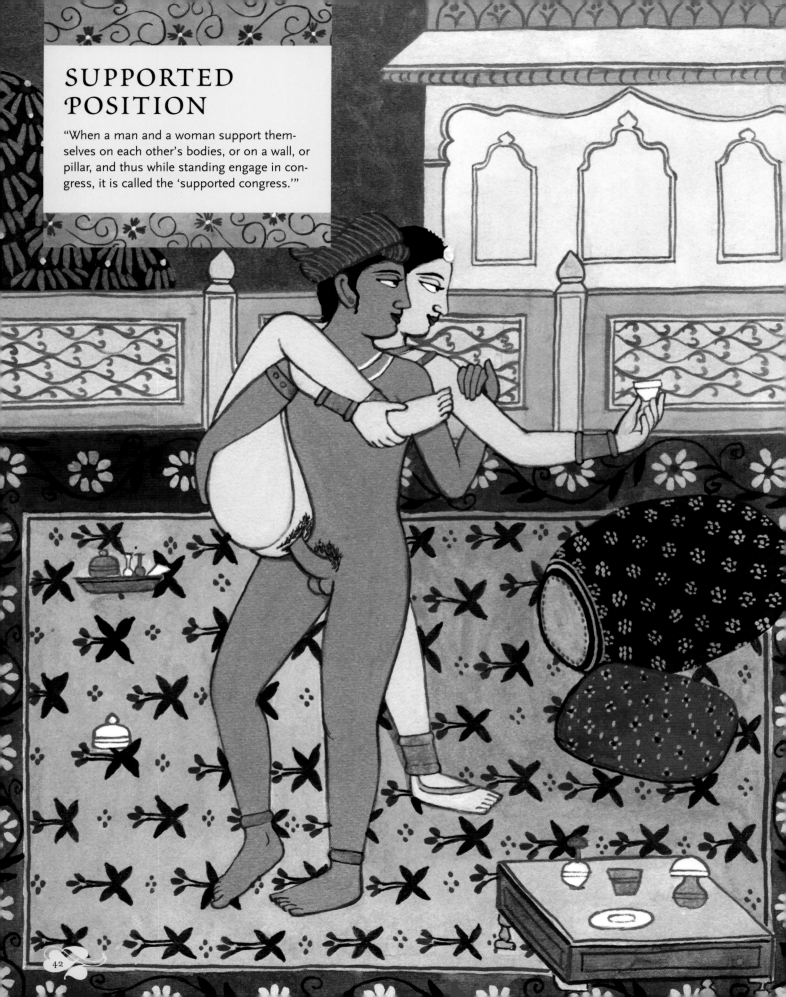

SUPPORTED
POSITION

"When a man and a woman support themselves on each other's bodies, or on a wall, or pillar, and thus while standing engage in congress, it is called the 'supported congress.'"

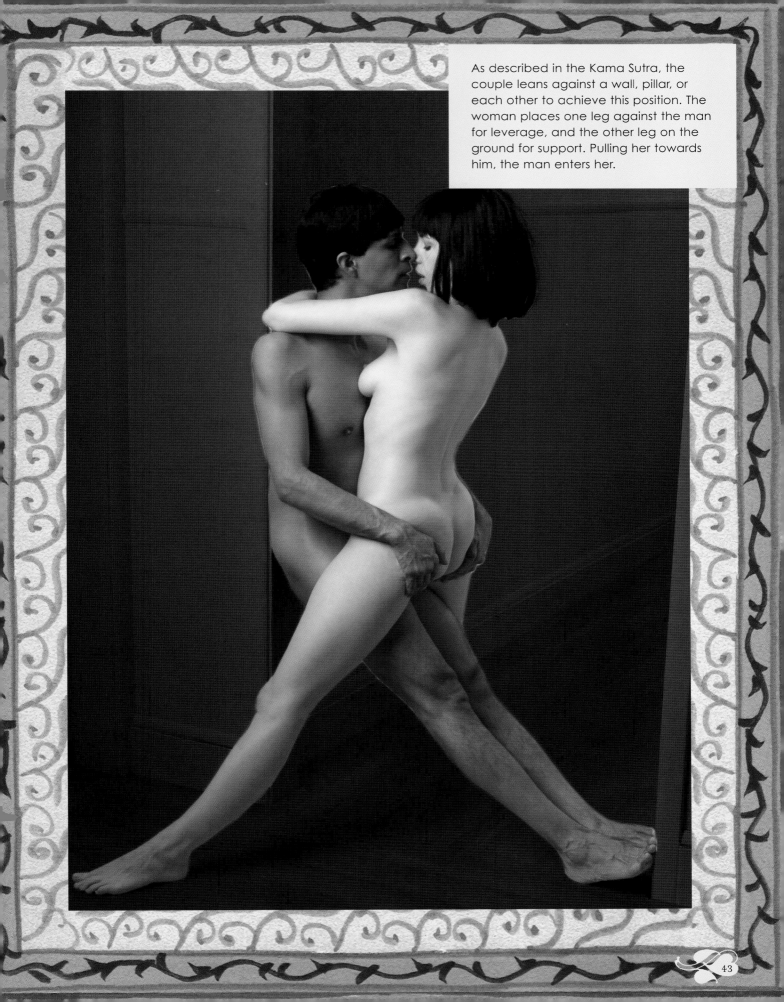

As described in the Kama Sutra, the couple leans against a wall, pillar, or each other to achieve this position. The woman places one leg against the man for leverage, and the other leg on the ground for support. Pulling her towards him, the man enters her.

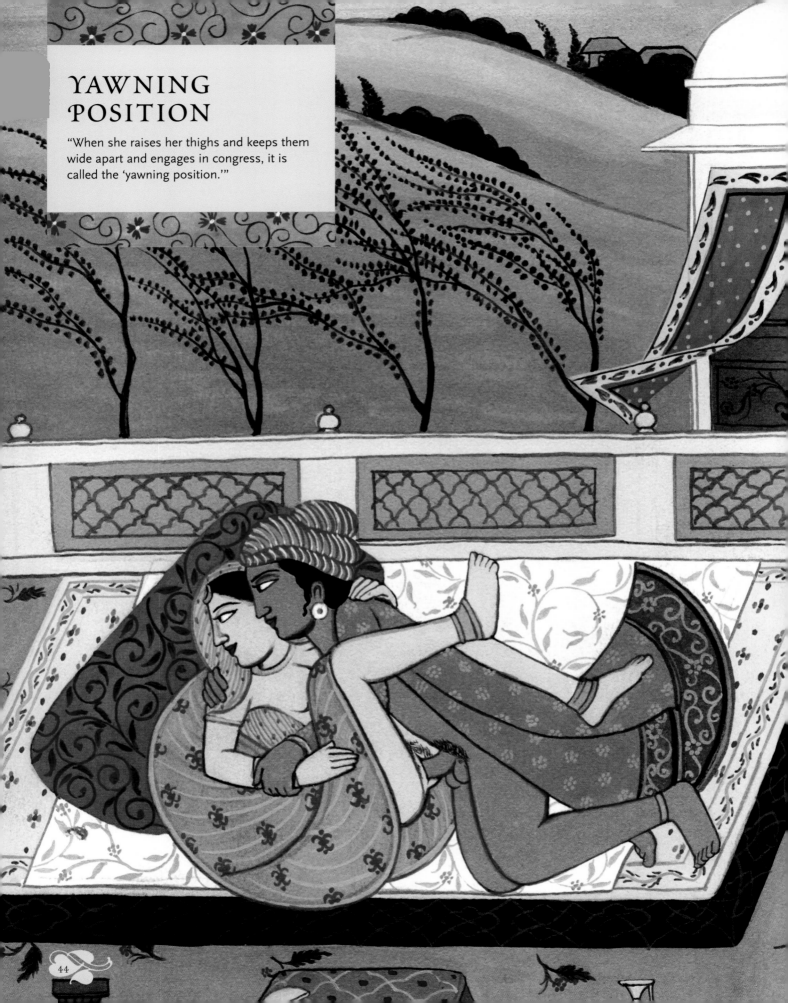

YAWNING
POSITION

"When she raises her thighs and keeps them wide apart and engages in congress, it is called the 'yawning position.'"

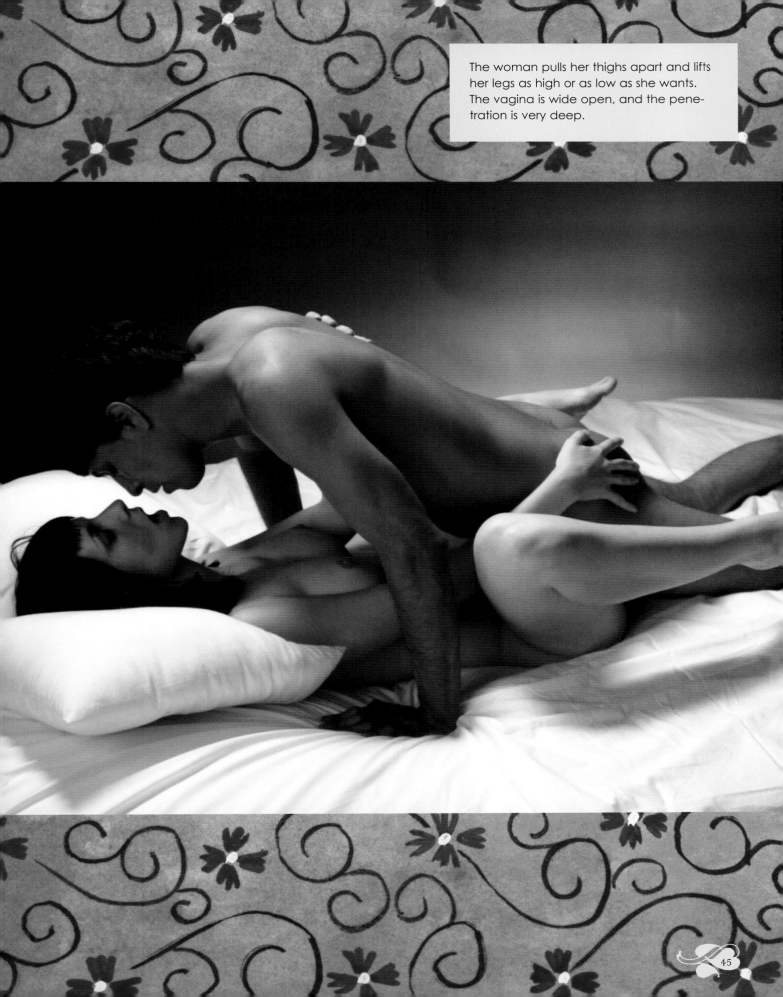

The woman pulls her thighs apart and lifts
her legs as high or as low as she wants.
The vagina is wide open, and the penetration is very deep.

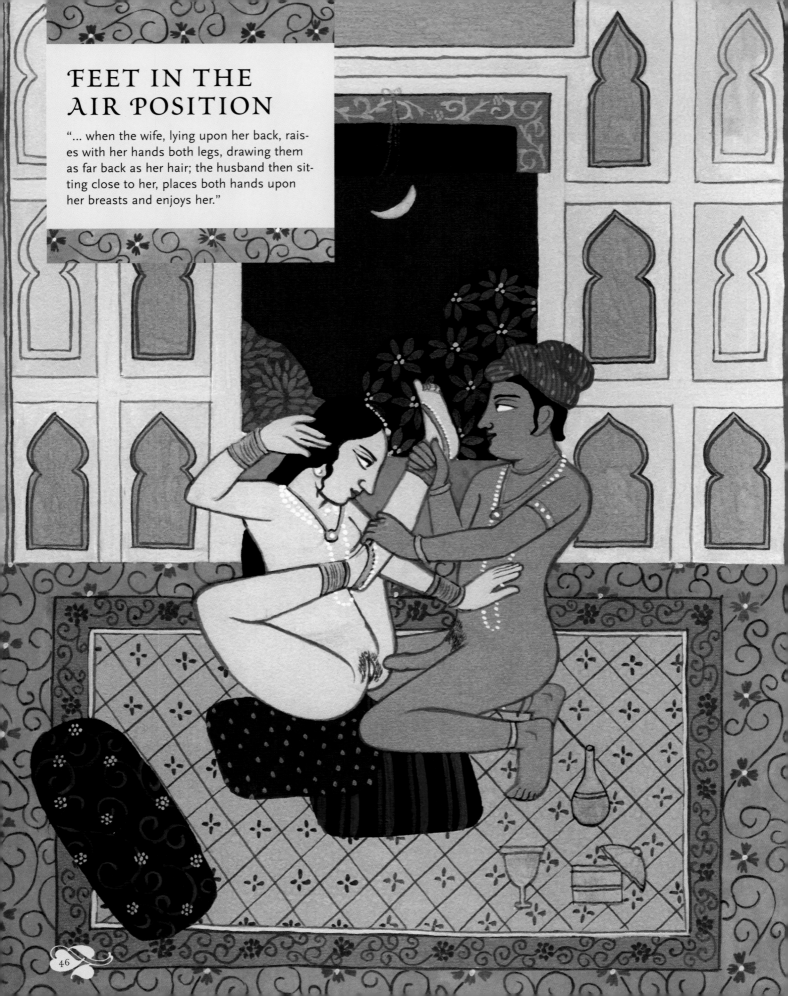

FEET IN THE
AIR POSITION

"... when the wife, lying upon her back, raises with her hands both legs, drawing them as far back as her hair; the husband then sitting close to her, places both hands upon her breasts and enjoys her."

The woman raises her legs and pulls them as far back as is comfortable. The man can hold her ankles for support and, kneeling in front of her, enter his lover.

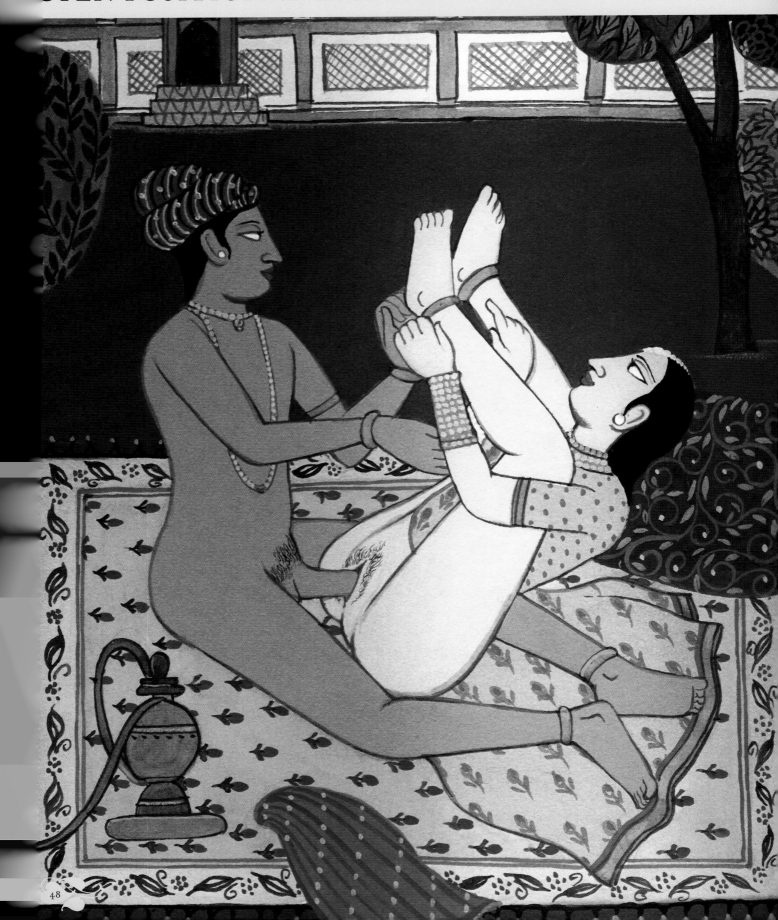

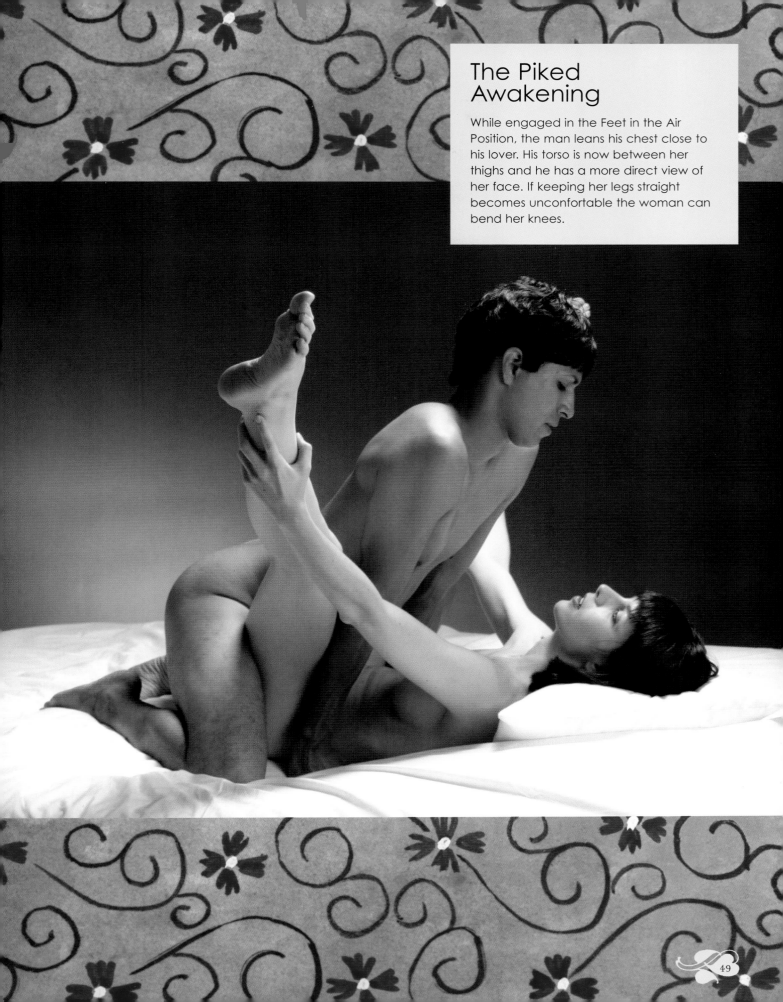

The Piked Awakening

While engaged in the Feet in the Air Position, the man leans his chest close to his lover. His torso is now between her thighs and he has a more direct view of her face. If keeping her legs straight becomes unconfortable the woman can bend her knees.

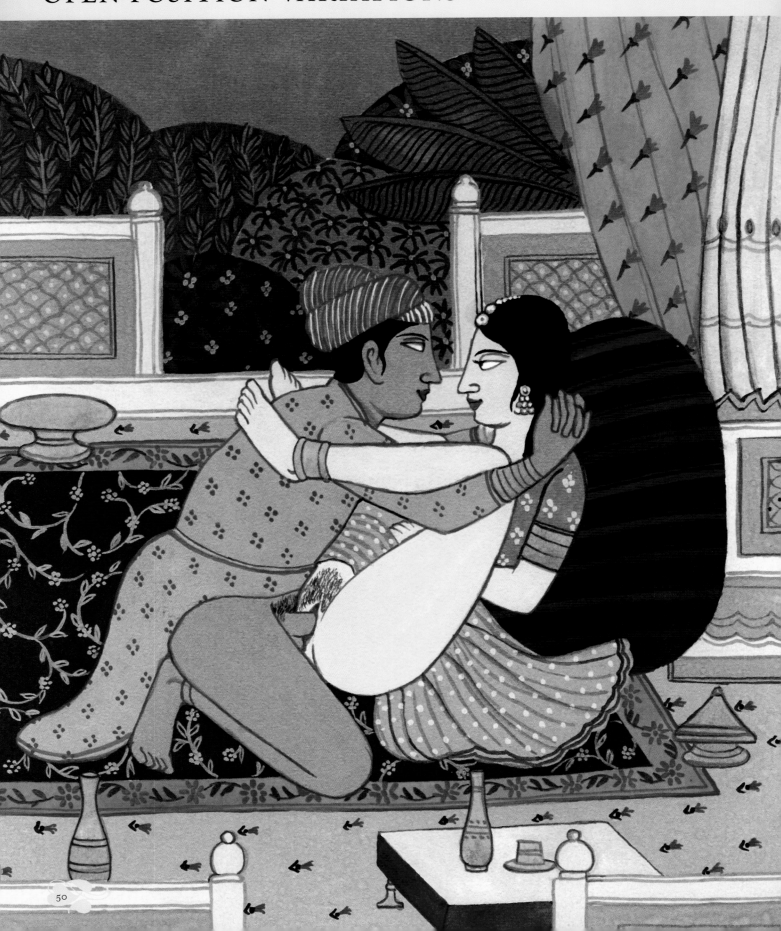

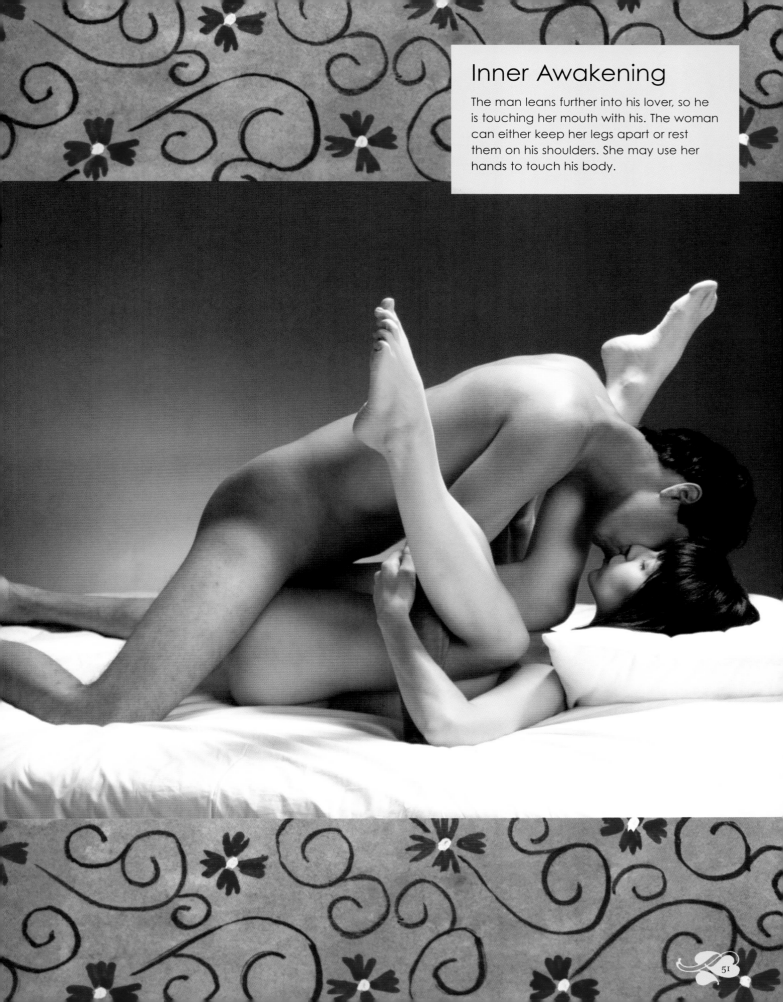

Inner Awakening

The man leans further into his lover, so he is touching her mouth with his. The woman can either keep her legs apart or rest them on his shoulders. She may use her hands to touch his body.

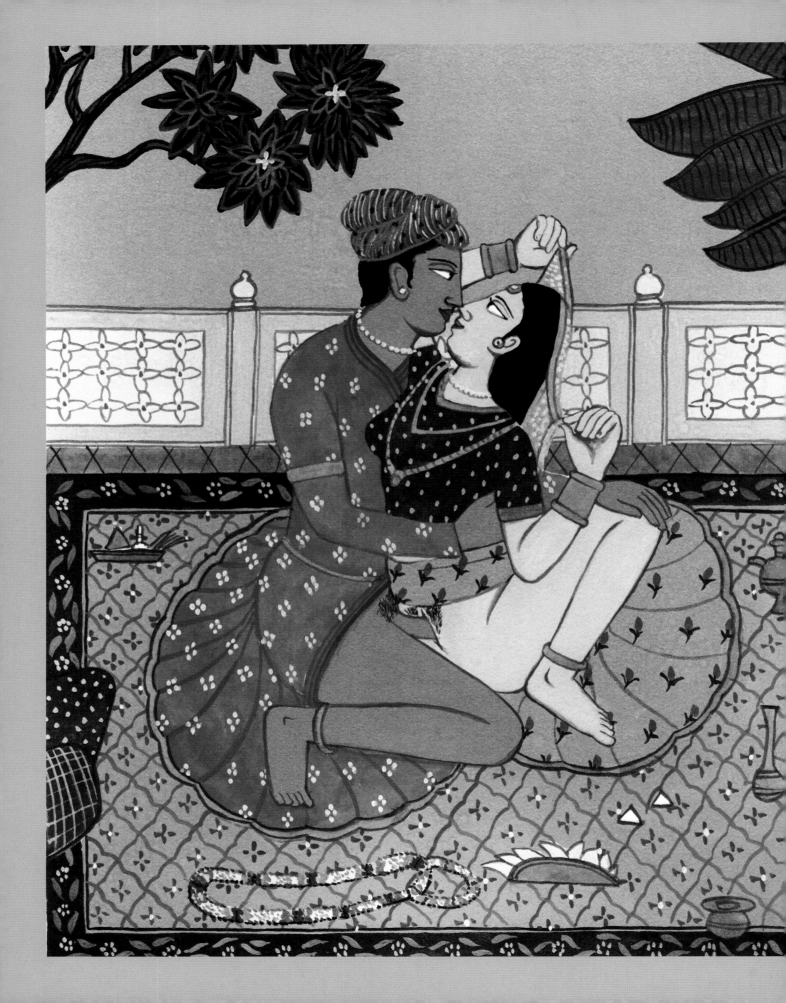

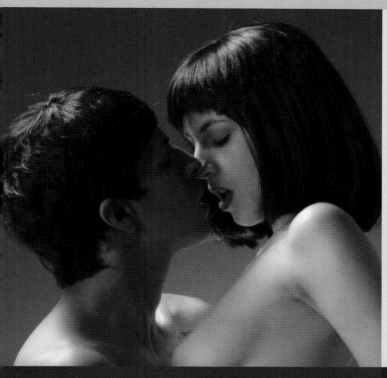

KISSING

Kissing is the beginning of intimacy, the introduction of desire, and a preview of the pleasure to come. Often described as the most intimate thing that can happen between two people, kissing is an integral part of the *Kama Sutra*, and it should be equally as important in a relationship. Kissing will add a level of closeness, as the couple will begin to understand the movement of each other's bodies and how he or she likes to be kissed.

Vatsyayana understood the importance of the kiss, and dedicated an entire chapter to it. He writes, "Kissing is of four kinds: moderate, contracted, pressed, and soft, according to the different parts of the body which are kissed, for different kinds of kisses are appropriate for different parts of the body." The lovers should take care to note how their partner responds to each different type of kiss.

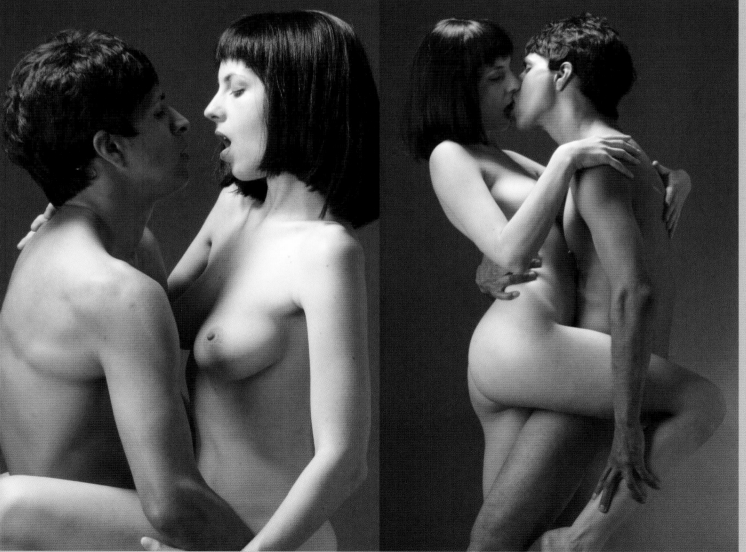

The *Kama Sutra* suggests, "The following are the places for kissing: the forehead, the eyes, the cheek, the throat, the bosom, the breasts, the lips, and the interior of the mouth." Before engaging in sex, the couple can spend time kissing each other in the various places mentioned in the *Kama Sutra*. The man can kiss the woman's breasts tenderly and the woman can press her lips against her partner's, as is instructed by Vatsyayana. This will bring the two together, and create an atmosphere of intimacy before the actual act begins.

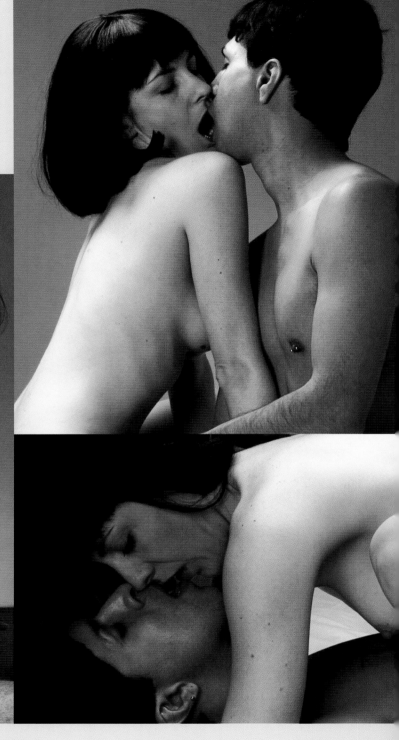

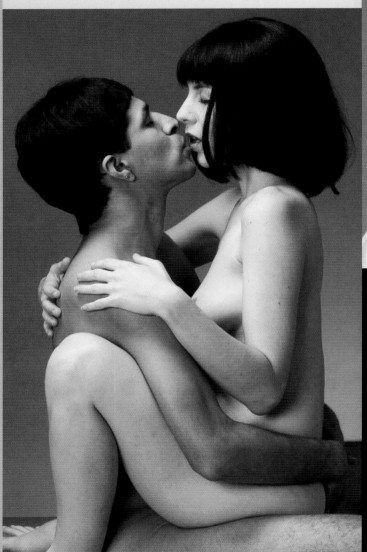

"KISSING CAN BE INTIMATE OR PLAYFUL, BUT IT IS ALMOST ALWAYS MAGICAL."

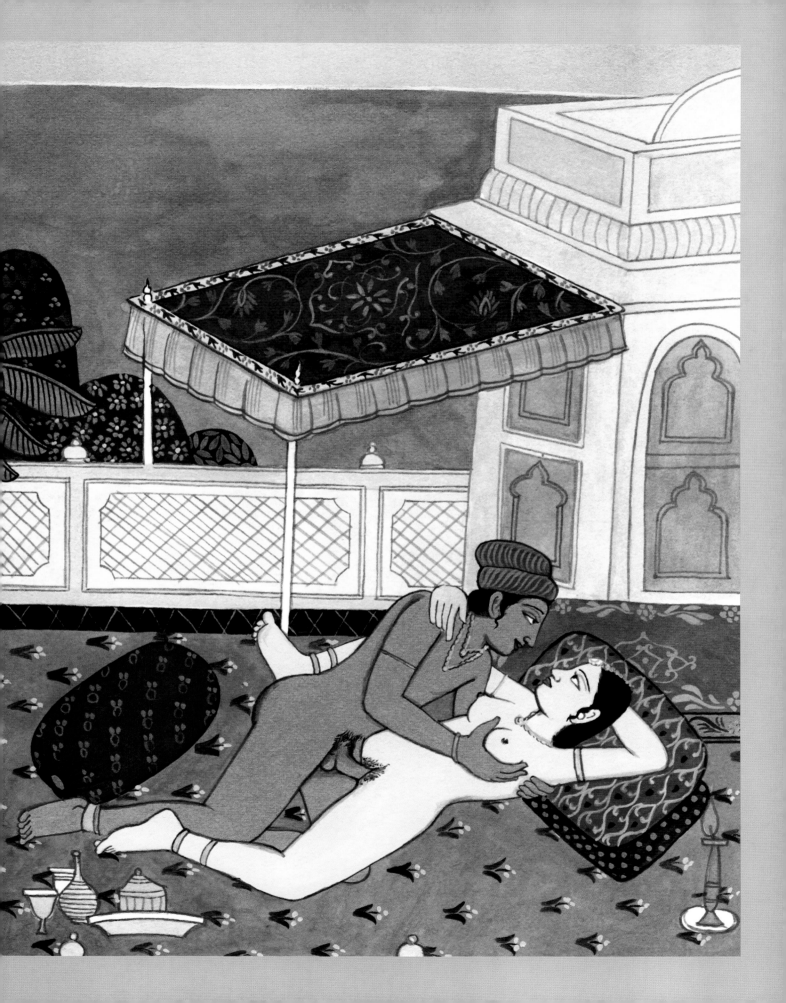

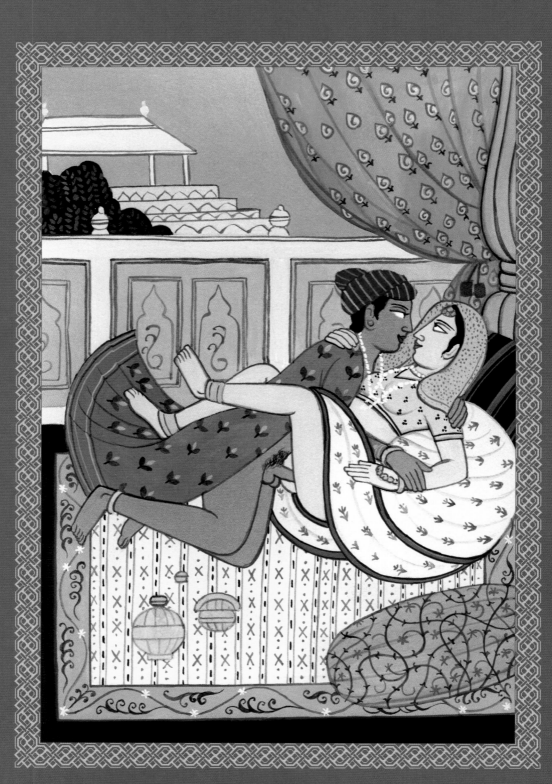

3
RISING
POSITIONS

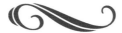

The rising positions are for couples who enjoy deep penetration and the intimacy that it brings. The woman is self confident in the movements of her body and her partner takes care to consider her needs and be open to her embraces.

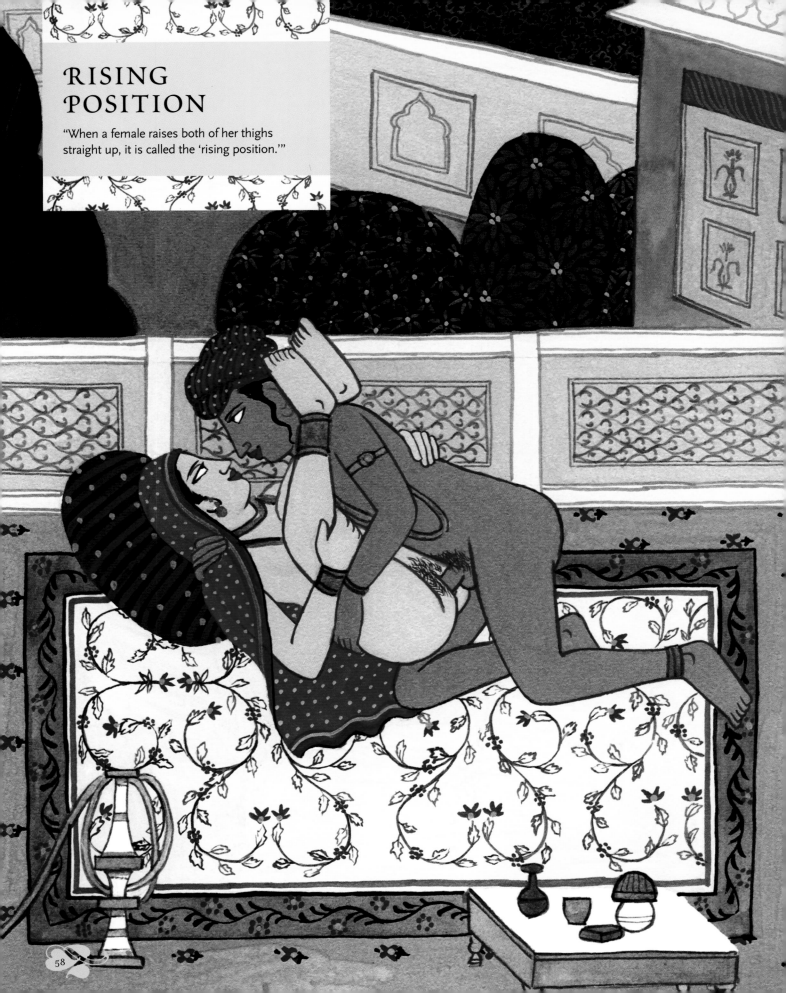

RISING POSITION

"When a female raises both of her thighs straight up, it is called the 'rising position.'"

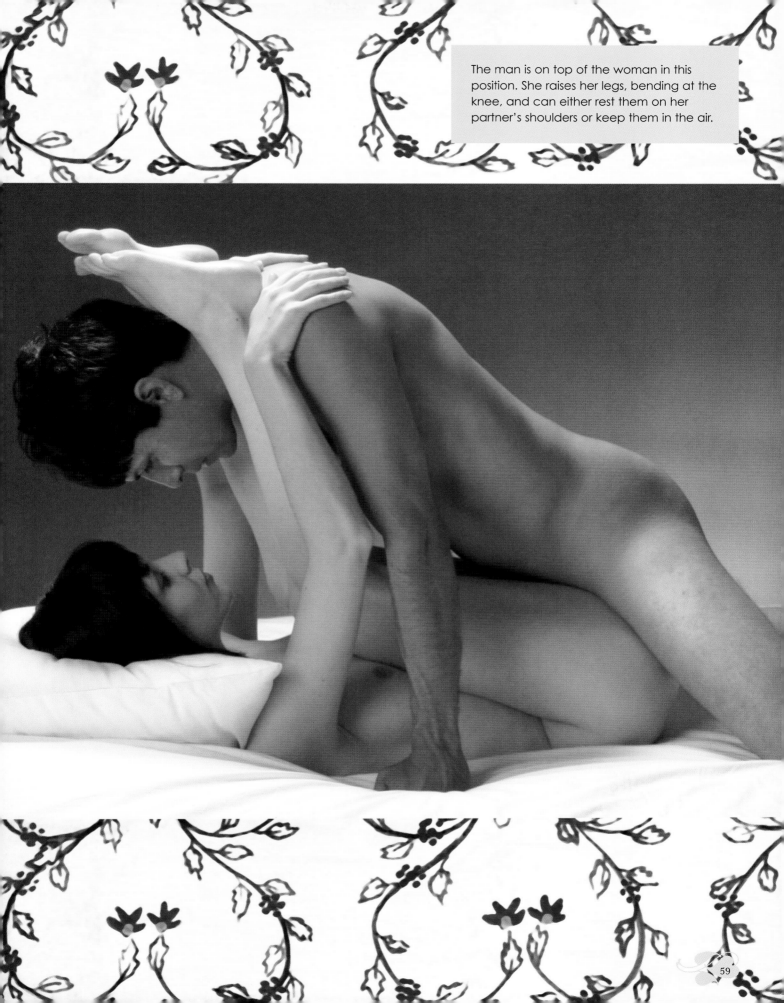

The man is on top of the woman in this position. She raises her legs, bending at the knee, and can either rest them on her partner's shoulders or keep them in the air.

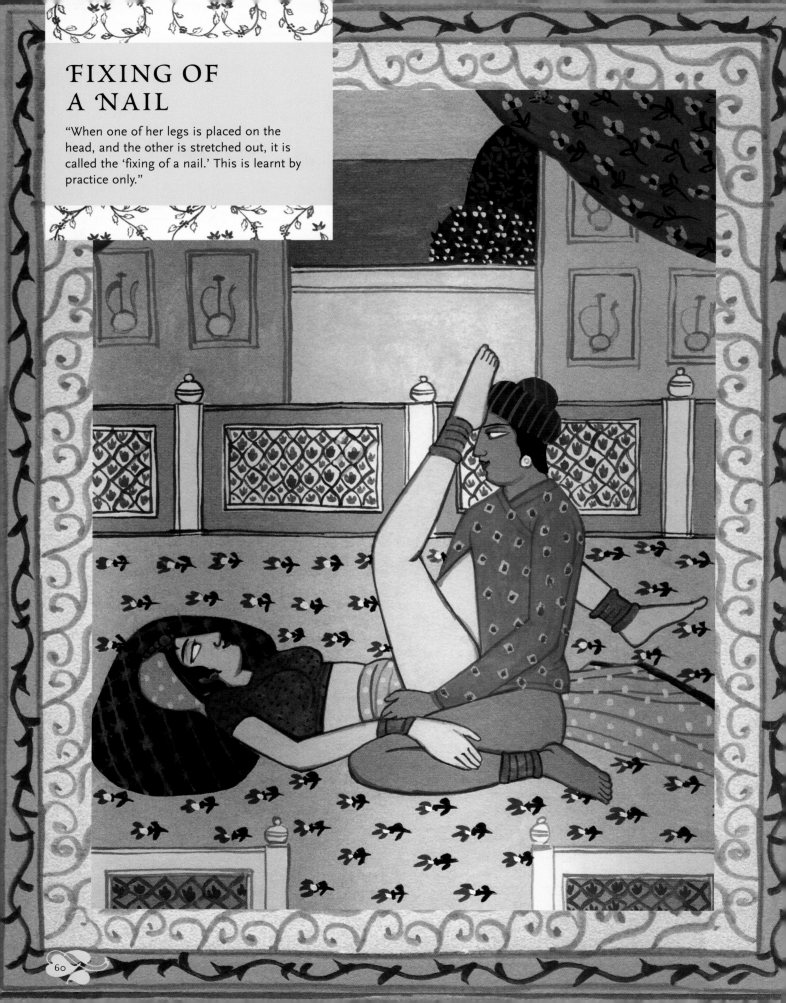

FIXING OF
A NAIL

"When one of her legs is placed on the head, and the other is stretched out, it is called the 'fixing of a nail.' This is learnt by practice only."

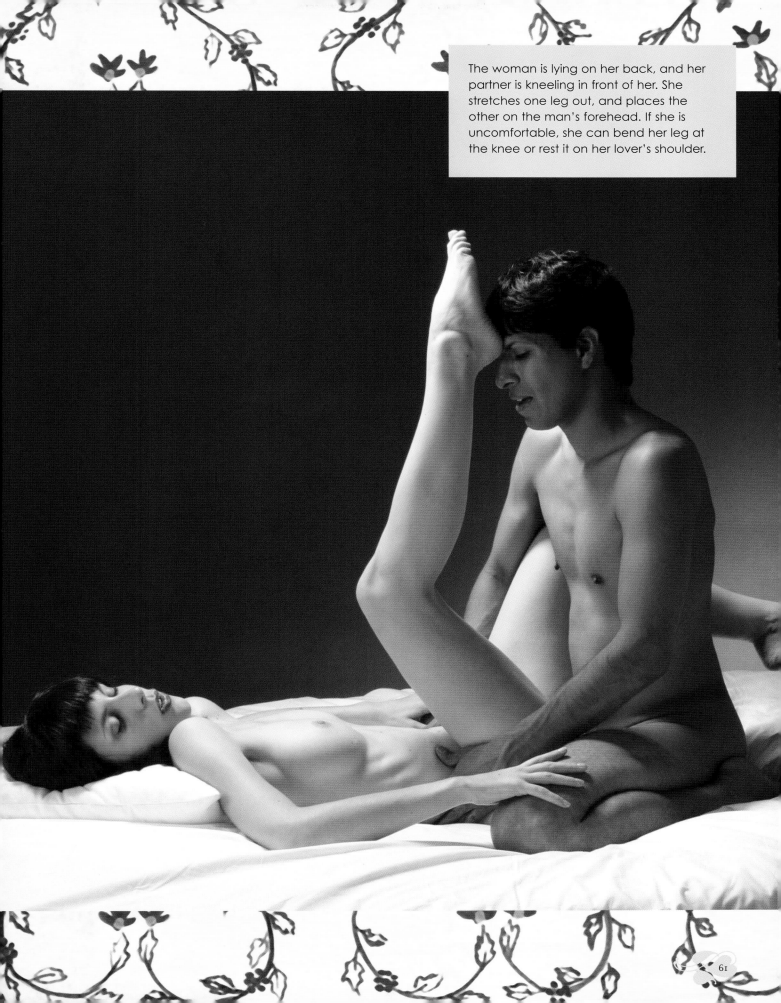

The woman is lying on her back, and her partner is kneeling in front of her. She stretches one leg out, and places the other on the man's forehead. If she is uncomfortable, she can bend her leg at the knee or rest it on her lover's shoulder.

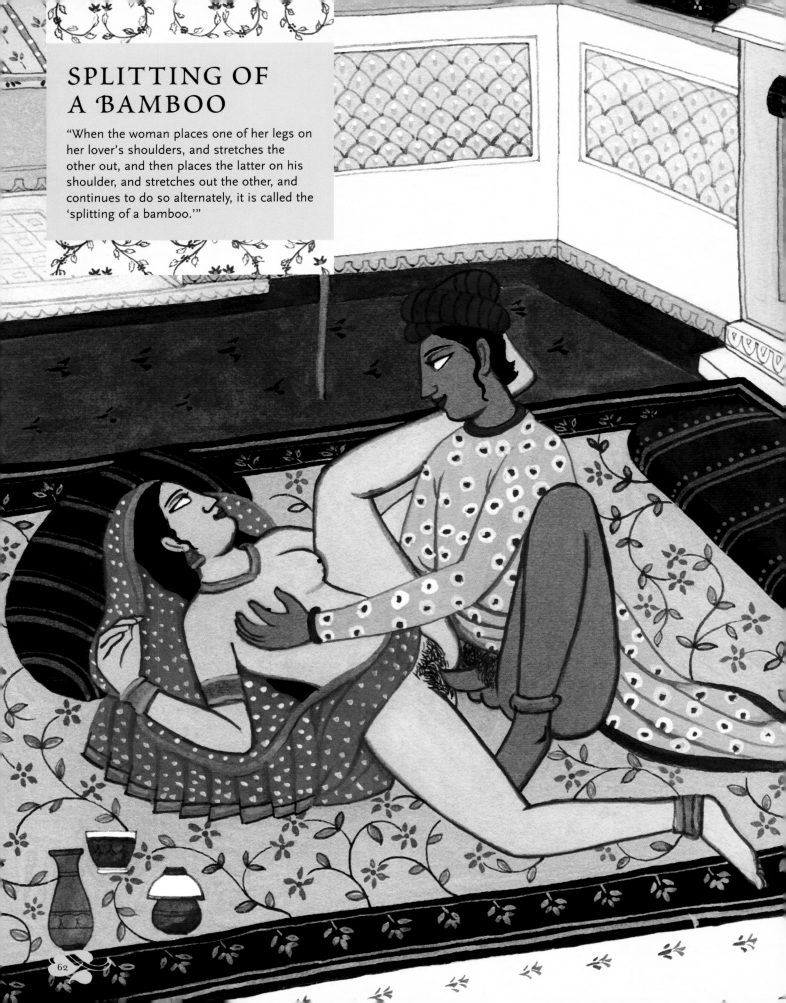

SPLITTING OF A BAMBOO

"When the woman places one of her legs on her lover's shoulders, and stretches the other out, and then places the latter on his shoulder, and stretches out the other, and continues to do so alternately, it is called the 'splitting of a bamboo.'"

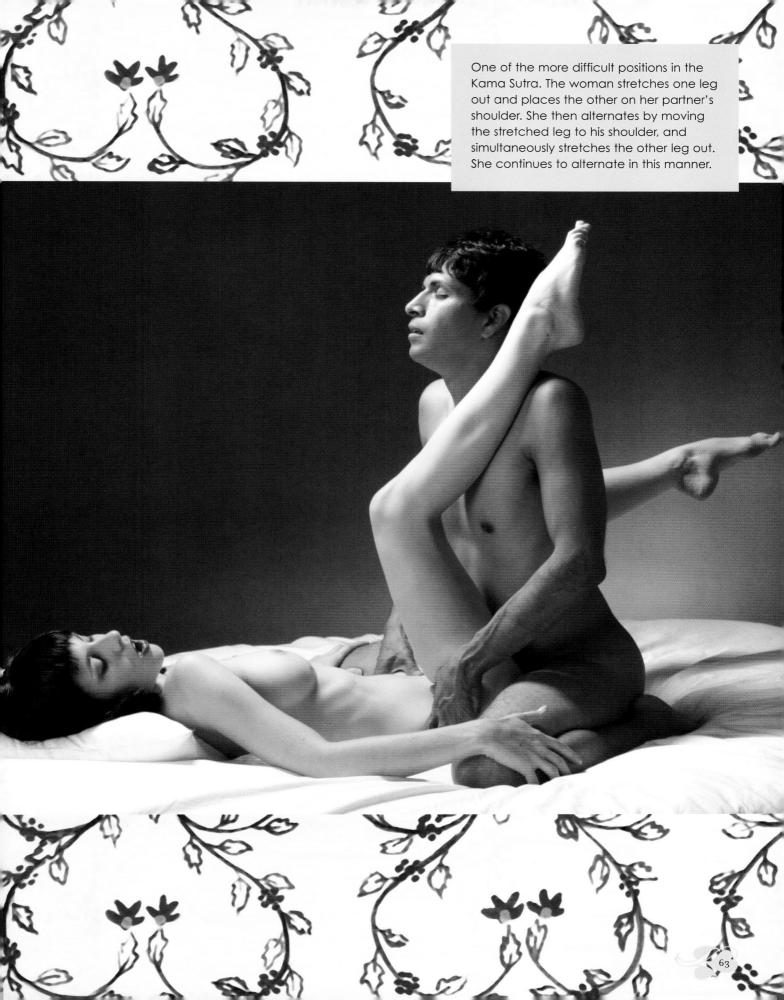

One of the more difficult positions in the Kama Sutra. The woman stretches one leg out and places the other on her partner's shoulder. She then alternates by moving the stretched leg to his shoulder, and simultaneously stretches the other leg out. She continues to alternate in this manner.

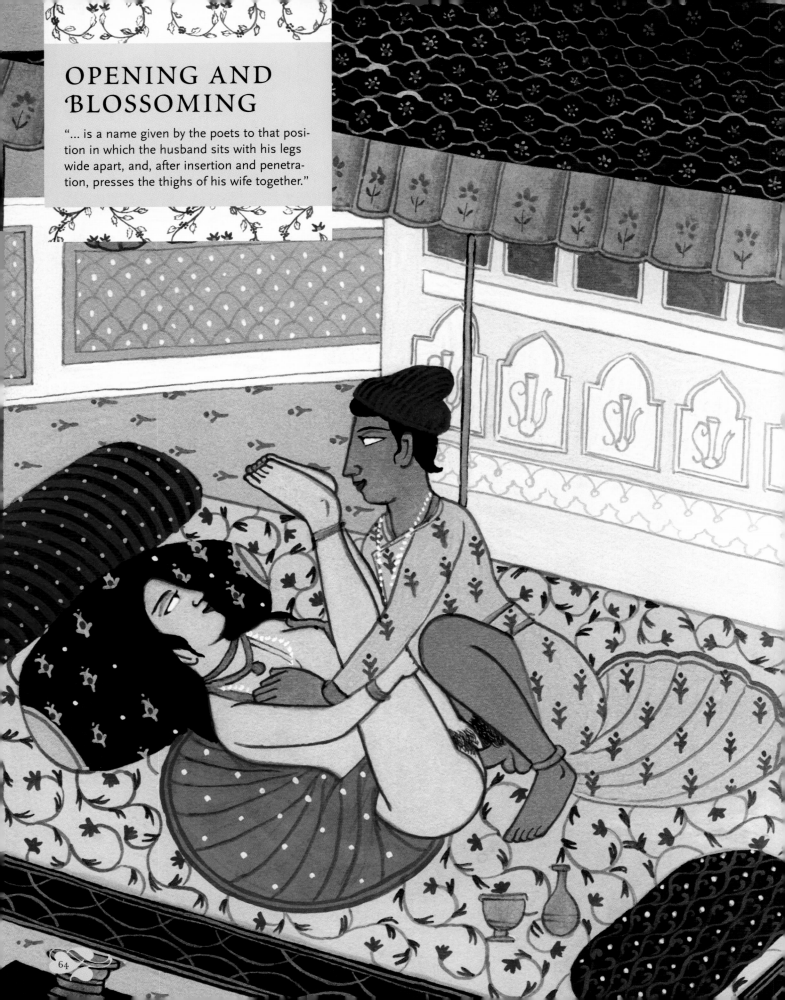

OPENING AND BLOSSOMING

"... is a name given by the poets to that position in which the husband sits with his legs wide apart, and, after insertion and penetration, presses the thighs of his wife together."

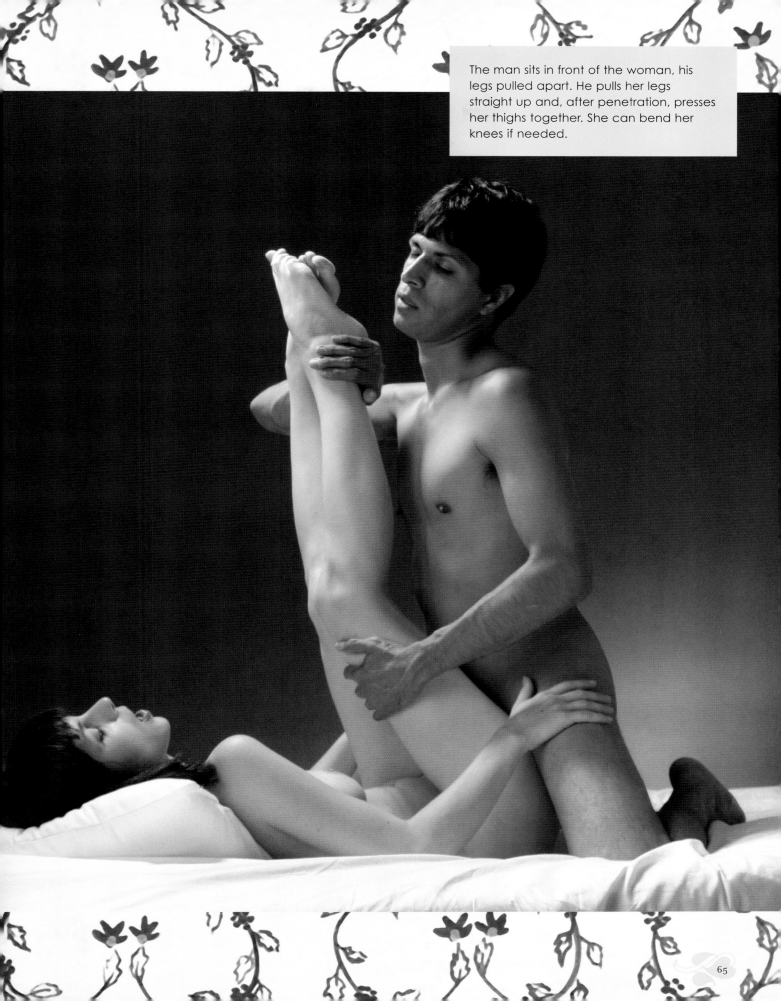

The man sits in front of the woman, his legs pulled apart. He pulls her legs straight up and, after penetration, presses her thighs together. She can bend her knees if needed.

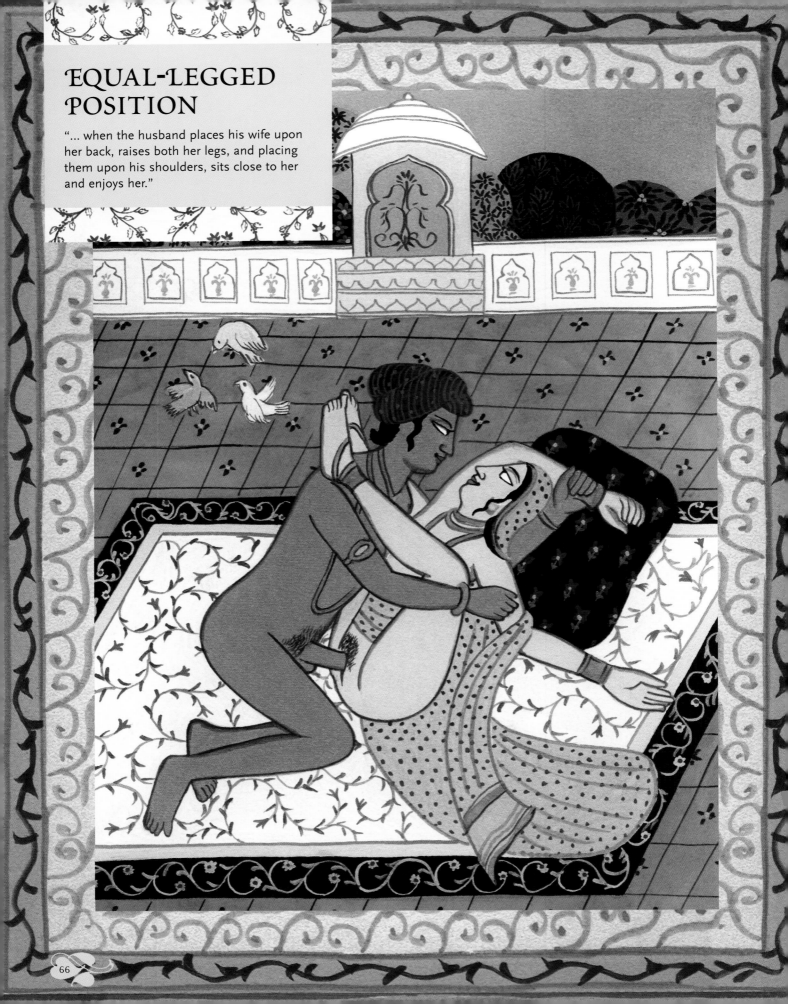

EQUAL-LEGGED POSITION

"… when the husband places his wife upon her back, raises both her legs, and placing them upon his shoulders, sits close to her and enjoys her."

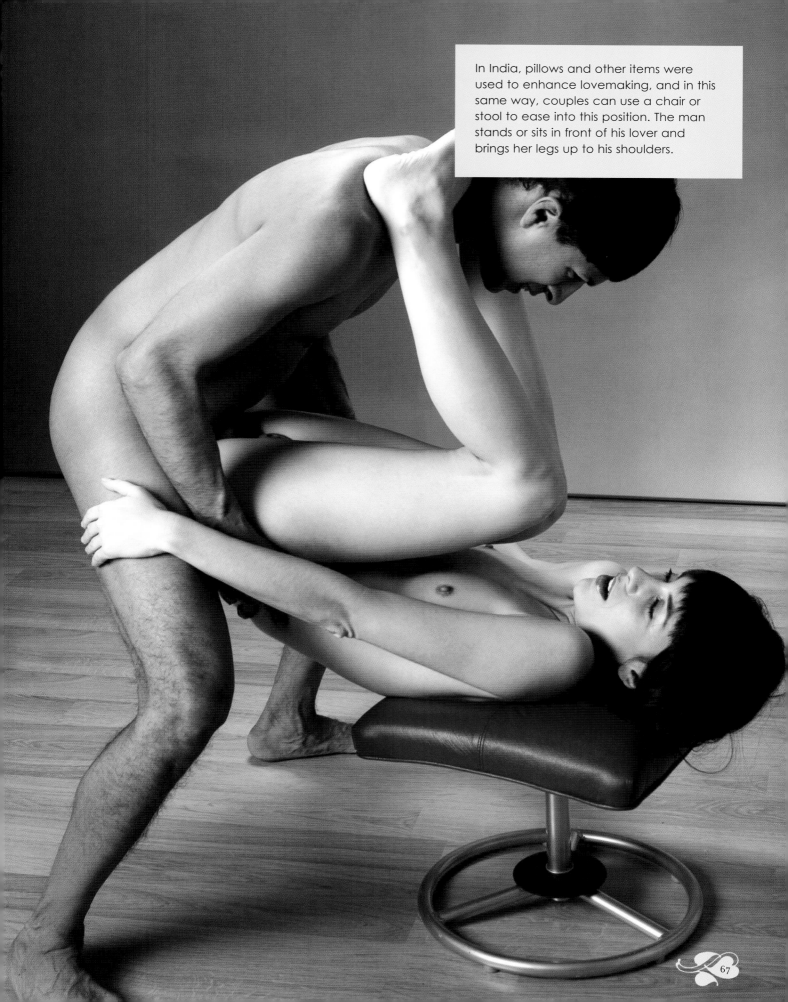

In India, pillows and other items were used to enhance lovemaking, and in this same way, couples can use a chair or stool to ease into this position. The man stands or sits in front of his lover and brings her legs up to his shoulders.

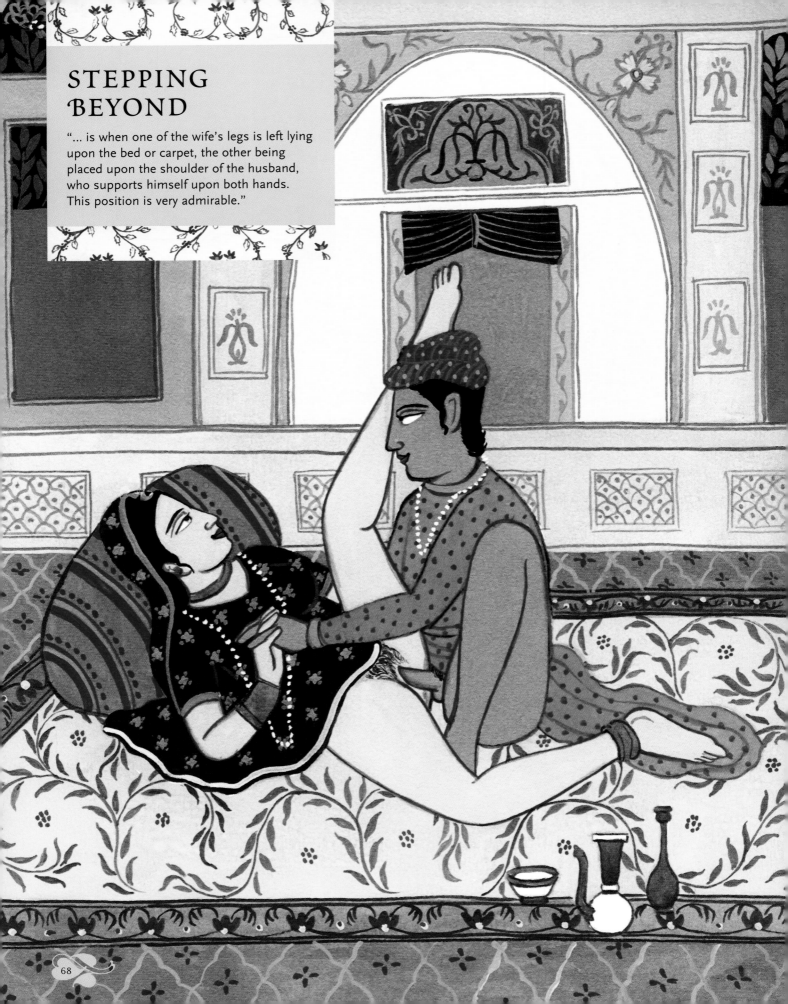

STEPPING BEYOND

"... is when one of the wife's legs is left lying upon the bed or carpet, the other being placed upon the shoulder of the husband, who supports himself upon both hands. This position is very admirable."

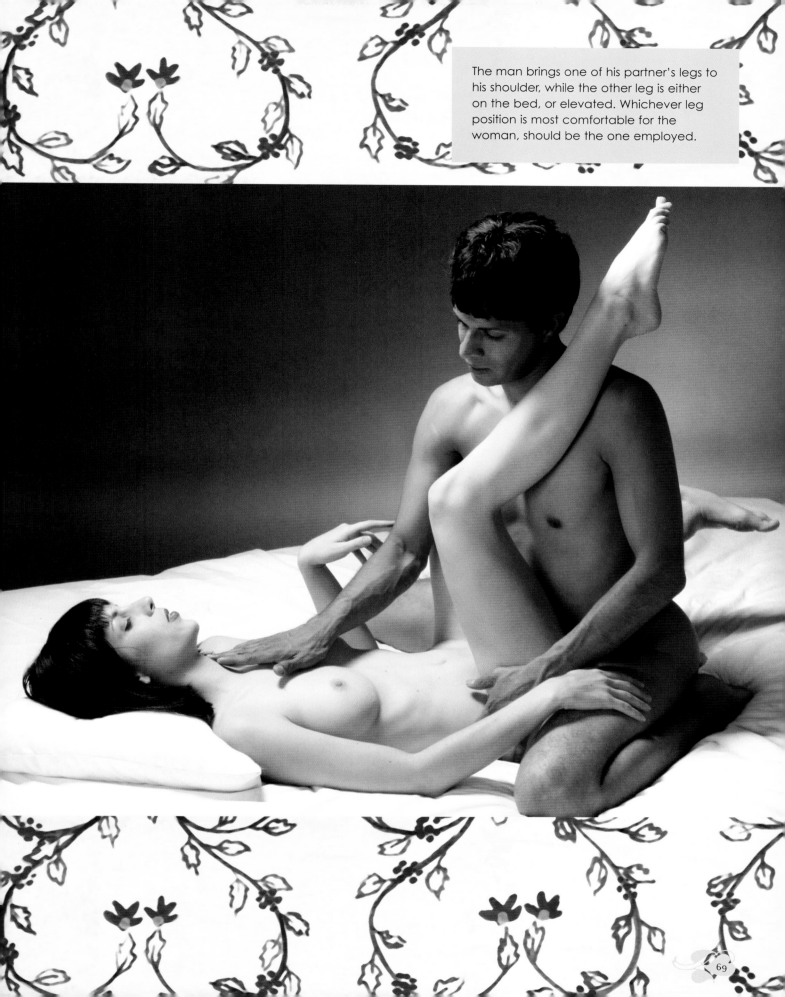

The man brings one of his partner's legs to his shoulder, while the other leg is either on the bed, or elevated. Whichever leg position is most comfortable for the woman, should be the one employed.

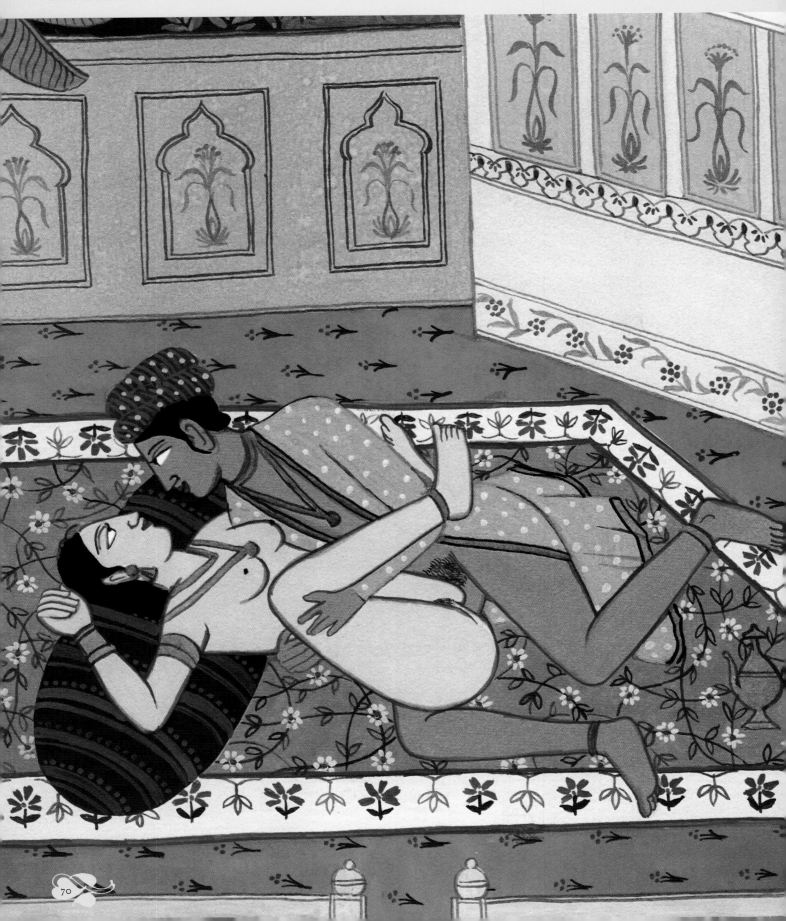

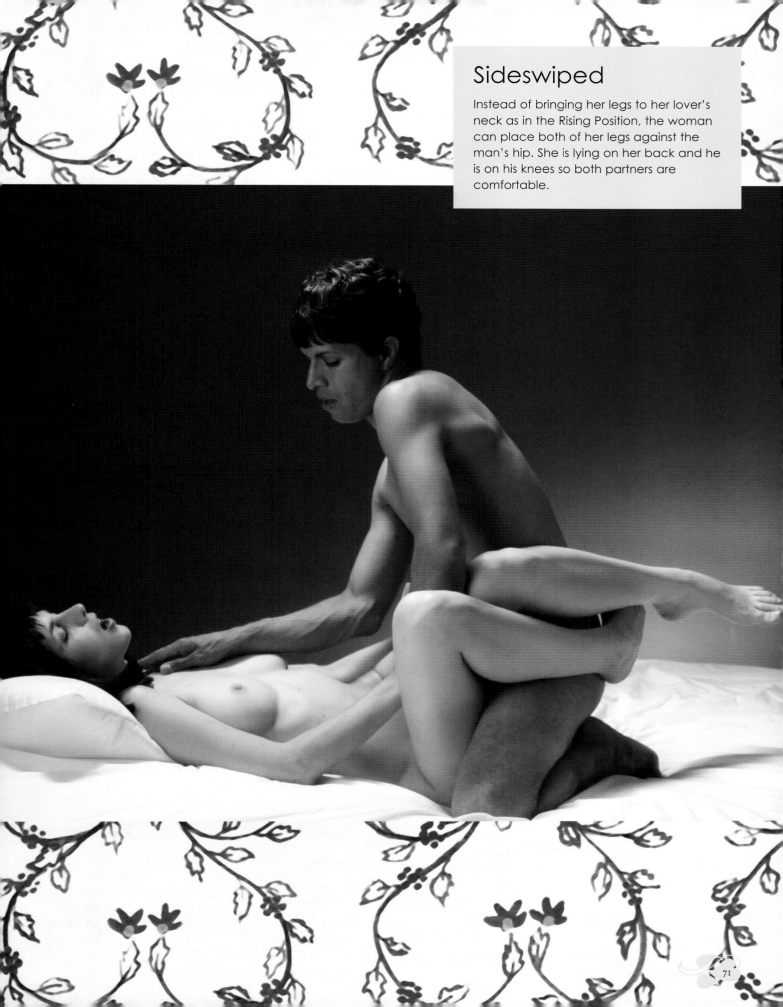

Sideswiped

Instead of bringing her legs to her lover's neck as in the Rising Position, the woman can place both of her legs against the man's hip. She is lying on her back and he is on his knees so both partners are comfortable.

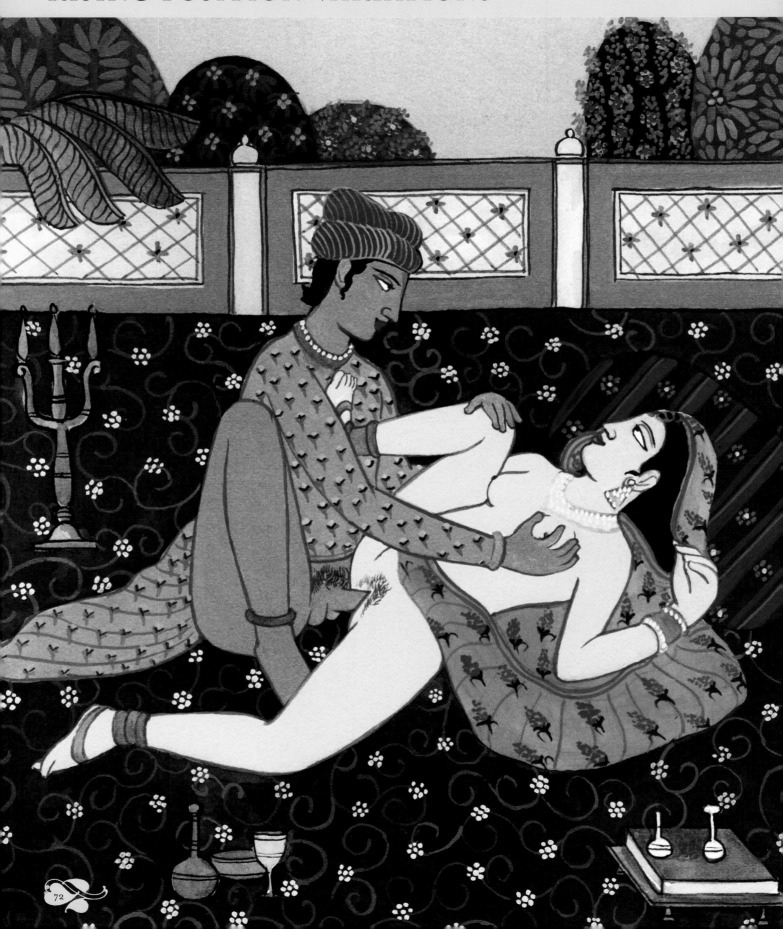

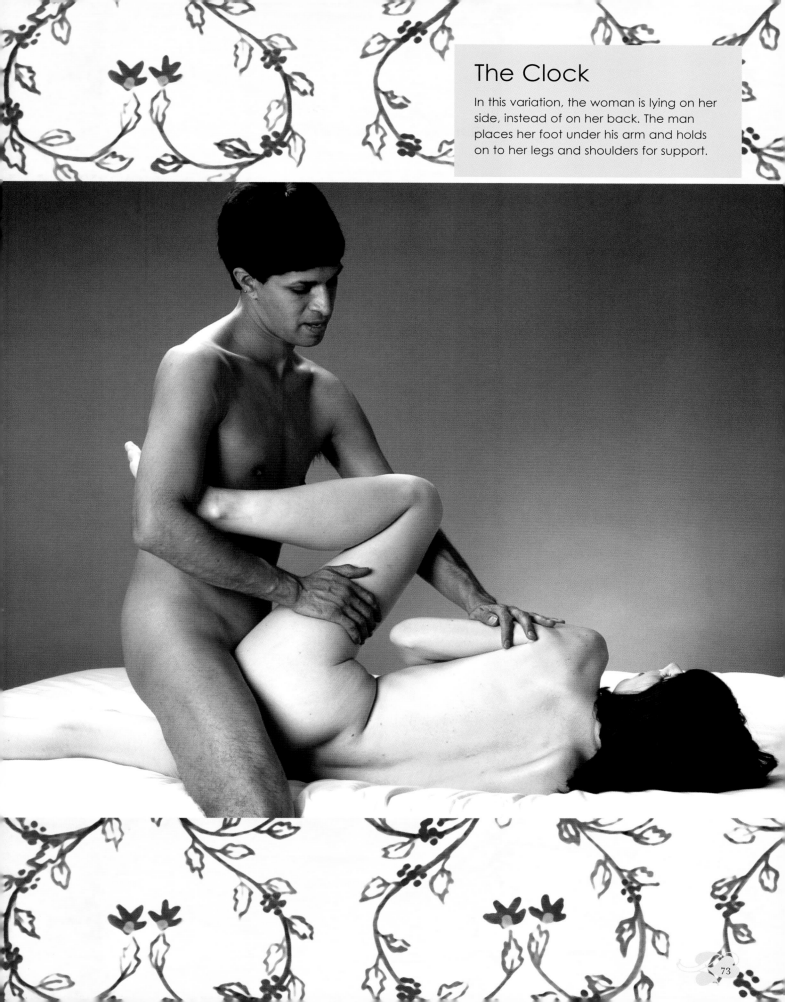

The Clock

In this variation, the woman is lying on her side, instead of on her back. The man places her foot under his arm and holds on to her legs and shoulders for support.

73

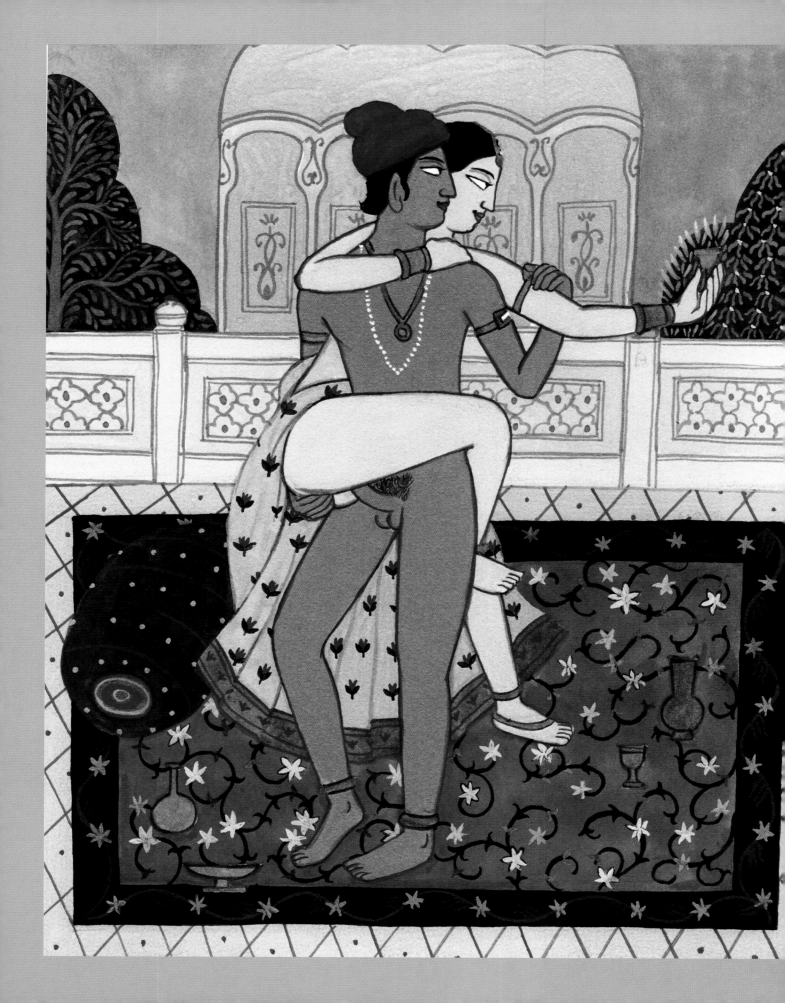

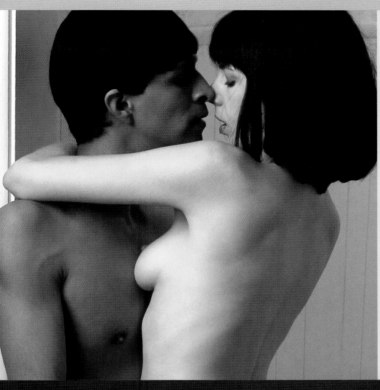

THE EMBRACE

Today, as in the time of Vatsyayana, embracing is much more than simply hugging. The *Kama Sutra* dedicates an entire chapter to the embrace, focusing on four different types: "Now the embrace which indicates the mutual love of a man and woman who have come together is of four kinds: touching, rubbing, piercing, pressing." Lovers can embrace each other around the neck, around the waist, or around the shoulders. Touching sends the signal that the couple is attracted to each other.

The embrace did not just mean hugging, but also embracing the breasts, pressing the other against a wall, or rubbing their bodies together. Vatsyayana writes, "When two lovers are walking slowly together, either in the dark, or in a place of public resort, or in a lonely place, and rub their bodies against each other, it is called a 'rubbing embrace.'"

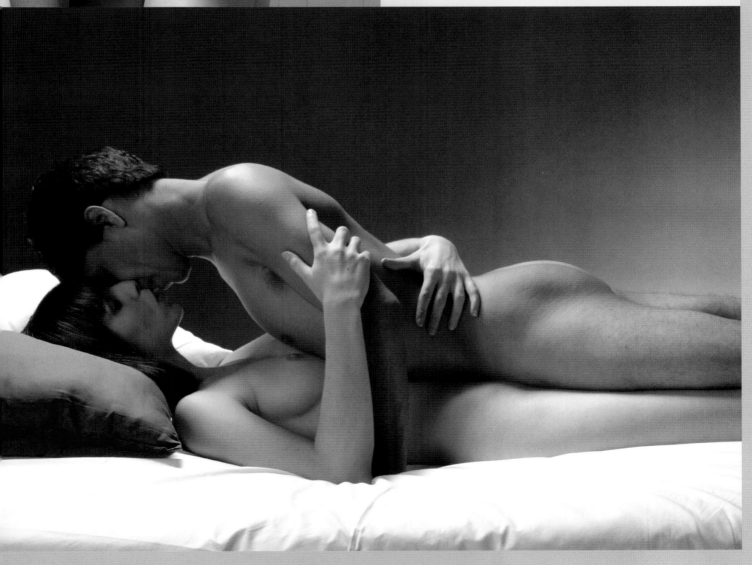

The *Kama Sutra* also stresses the importance of embracing during sex. "The Mixture of Sesamum Seed with Rice" in which the arms and thighs of the lovers are intertwined, and the "Mixture of Milk and Water," in which the lovers embrace while the woman sits on the man's lap, were intended to occur either right before, or during sex. Adding to the intimacy of the act, embracing also adds a sensuality that connects the lovers on many new levels.

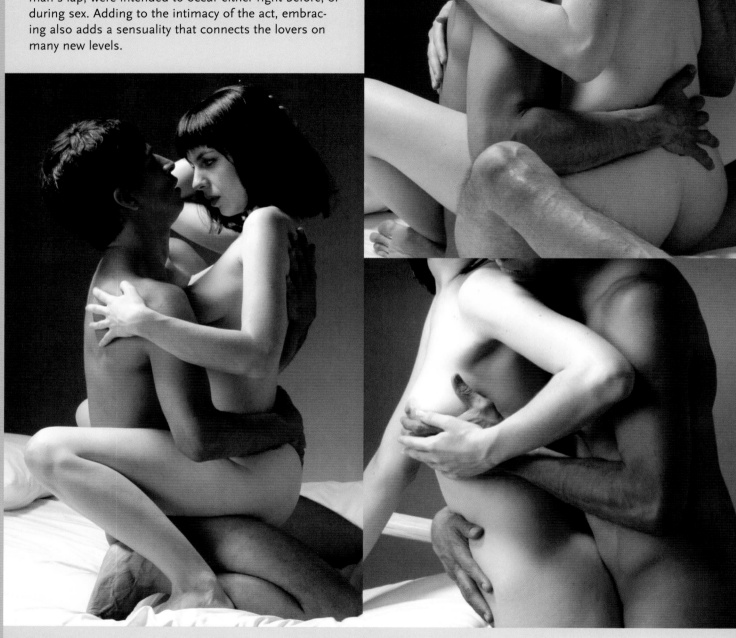

"WHAT OTHER FORM OF FOREPLAY CAN TAKE PLACE IN YOUR MOTHER'S KITCHEN? YOU CAN EMBRACE ANYWHERE."

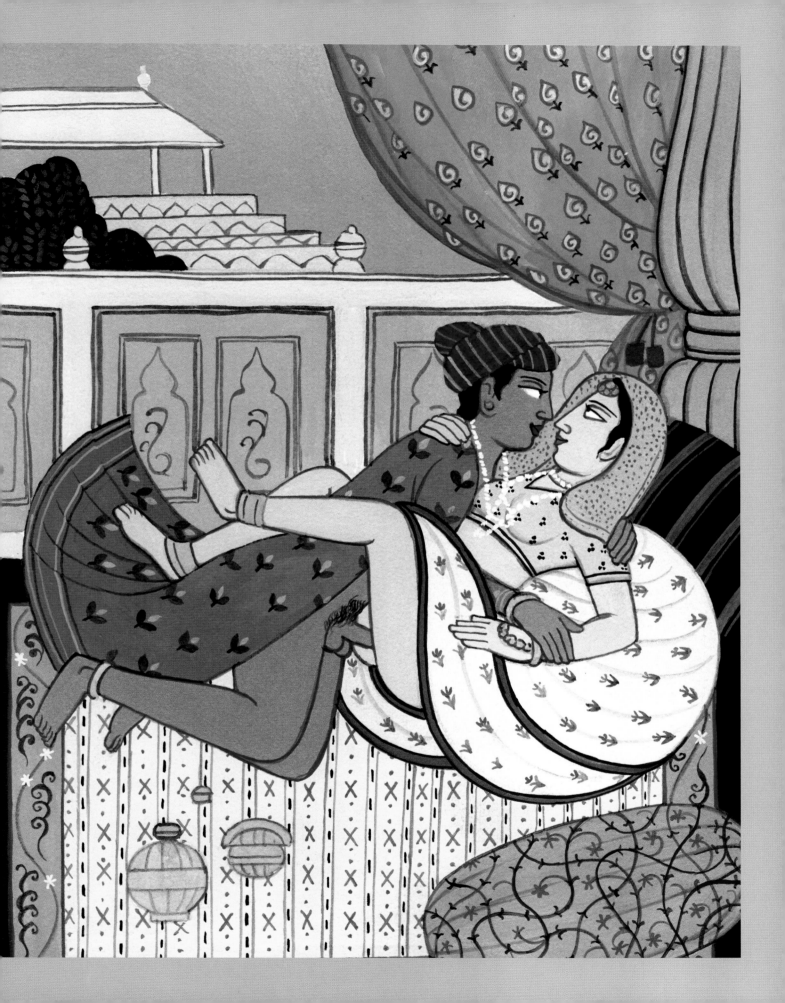

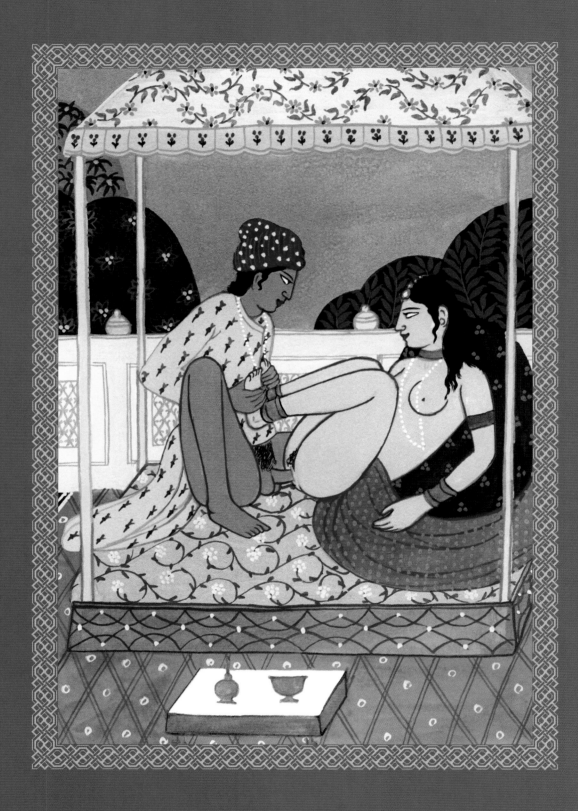

PRESSED POSITIONS

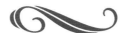

The man takes control in the Pressed Positions. He presses close to his lover, holding and guiding her body in sensual and intimate ways that will bring both of them pleasure.

CRAB'S POSITION

"When both the legs of the woman are contracted, and placed on her stomach, it is called the 'crab's position.'"

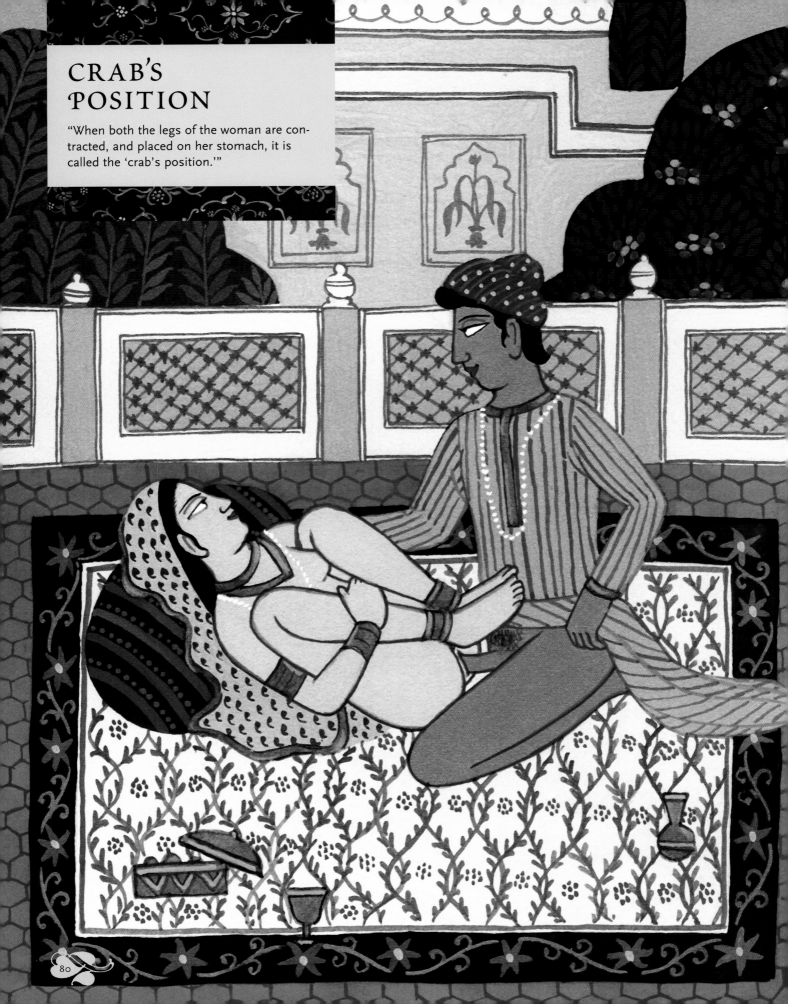

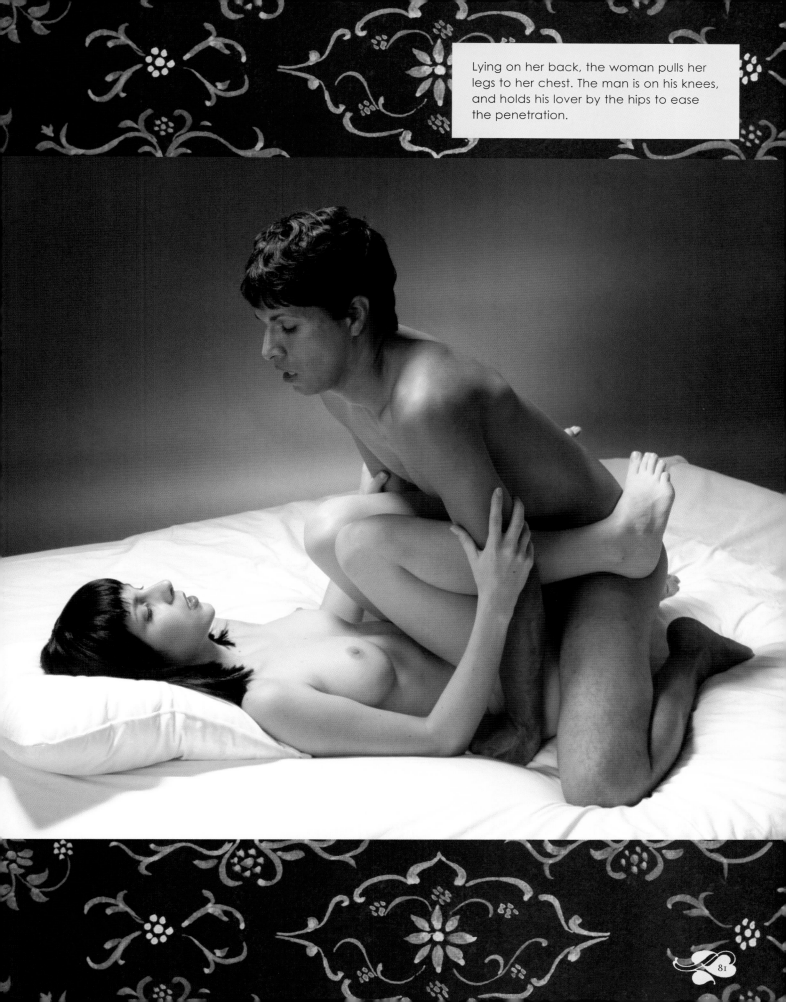

Lying on her back, the woman pulls her legs to her chest. The man is on his knees, and holds his lover by the hips to ease the penetration.

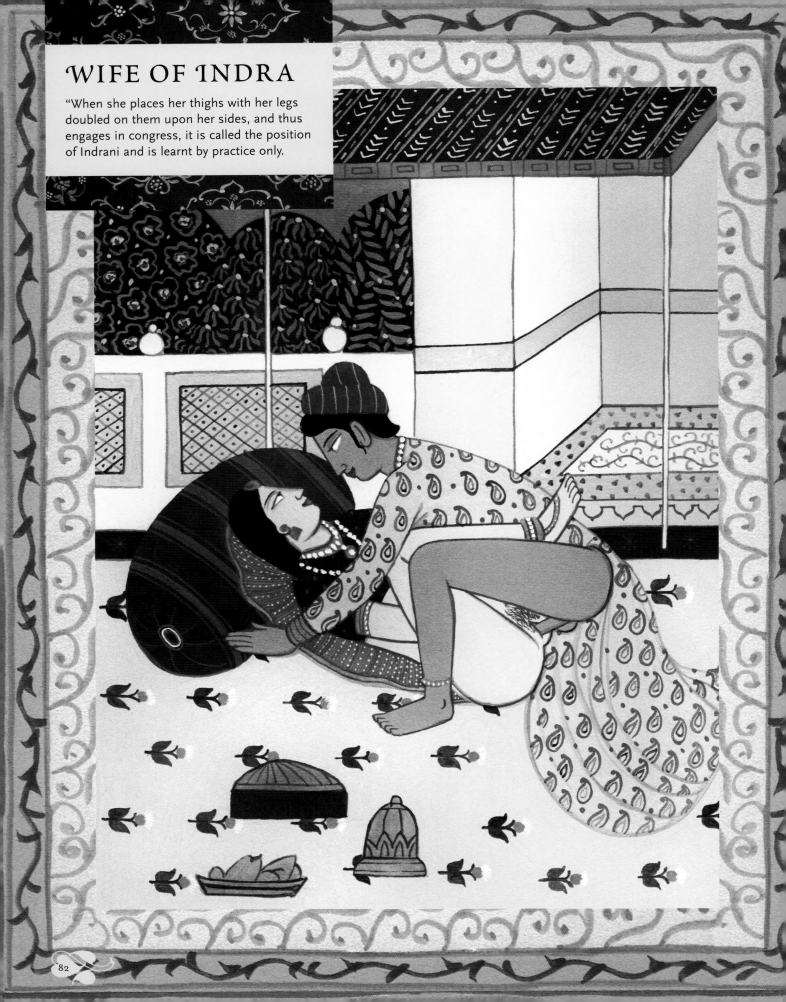

WIFE OF INDRA

"When she places her thighs with her legs doubled on them upon her sides, and thus engages in congress, it is called the position of Indrani and is learnt by practice only.

A slight variation of the Crab's position, the woman pulls her legs up so that her thighs are perpendicular to the bed. The man holds his lover's hips and leans in to kiss her breasts and stomach.

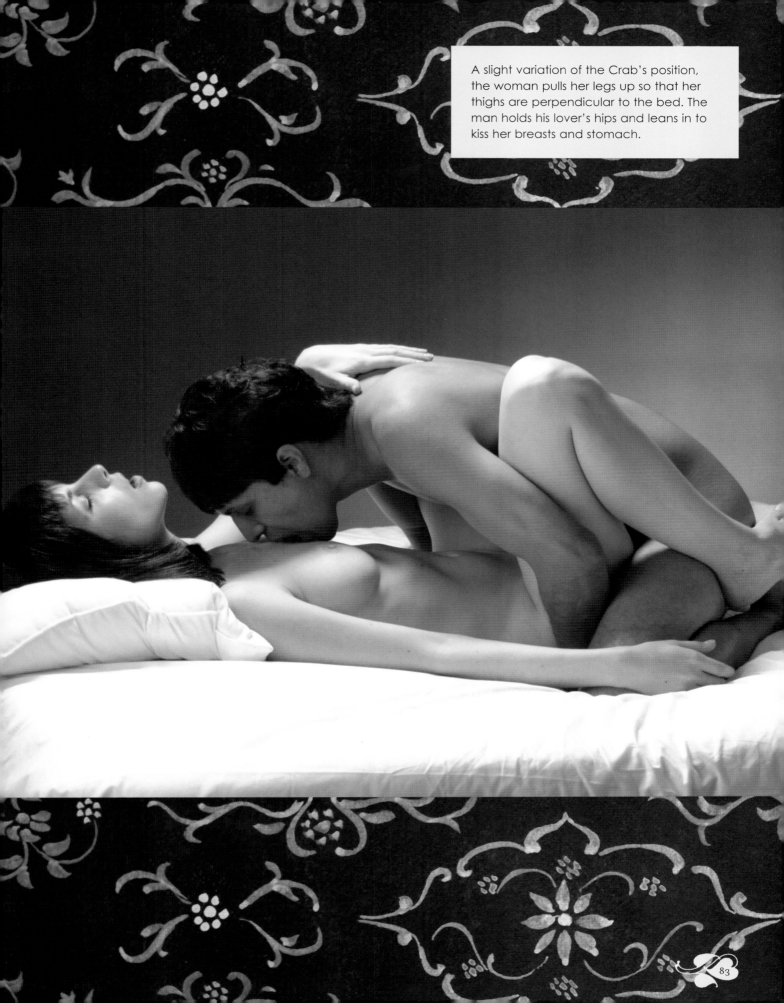

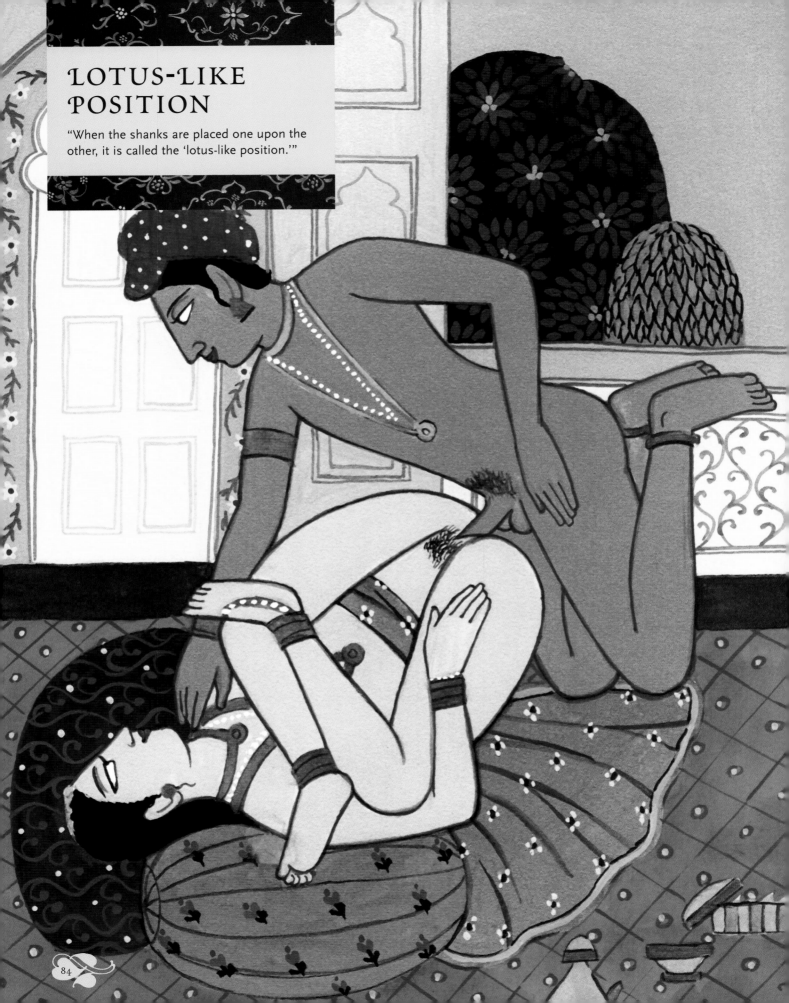

LOTUS-LIKE POSITION

"When the shanks are placed one upon the other, it is called the 'lotus-like position.'"

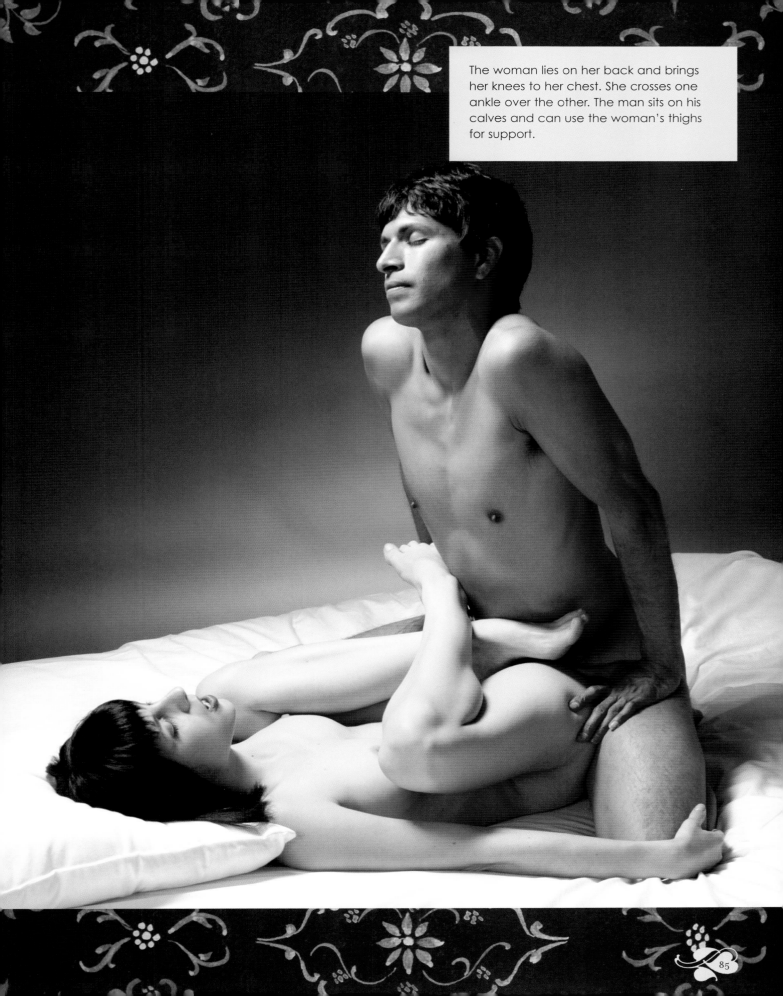

The woman lies on her back and brings her knees to her chest. She crosses one ankle over the other. The man sits on his calves and can use the woman's thighs for support.

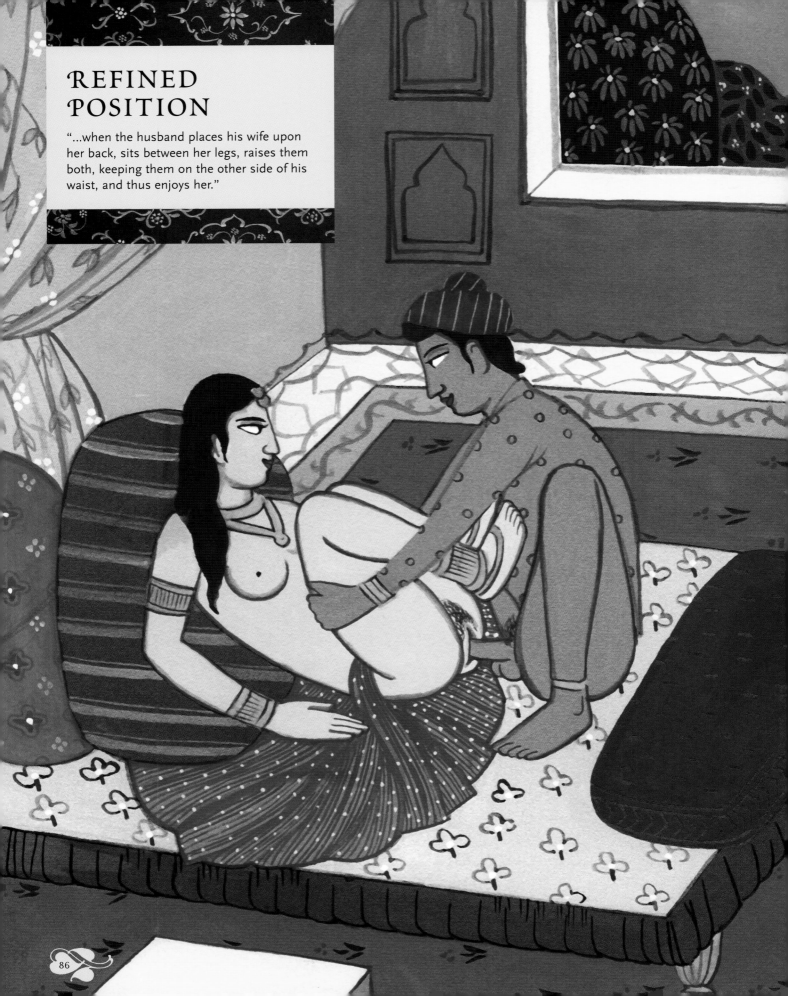

REFINED POSITION

"...when the husband places his wife upon her back, sits between her legs, raises them both, keeping them on the other side of his waist, and thus enjoys her."

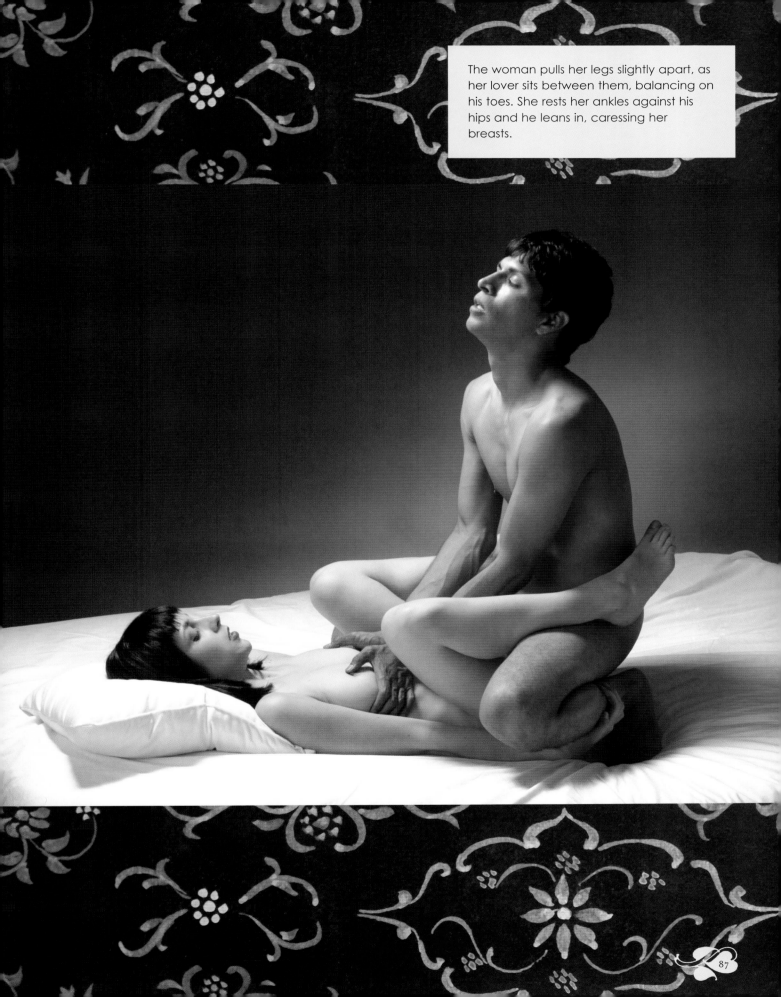

The woman pulls her legs slightly apart, as her lover sits between them, balancing on his toes. She rests her ankles against his hips and he leans in, caressing her breasts.

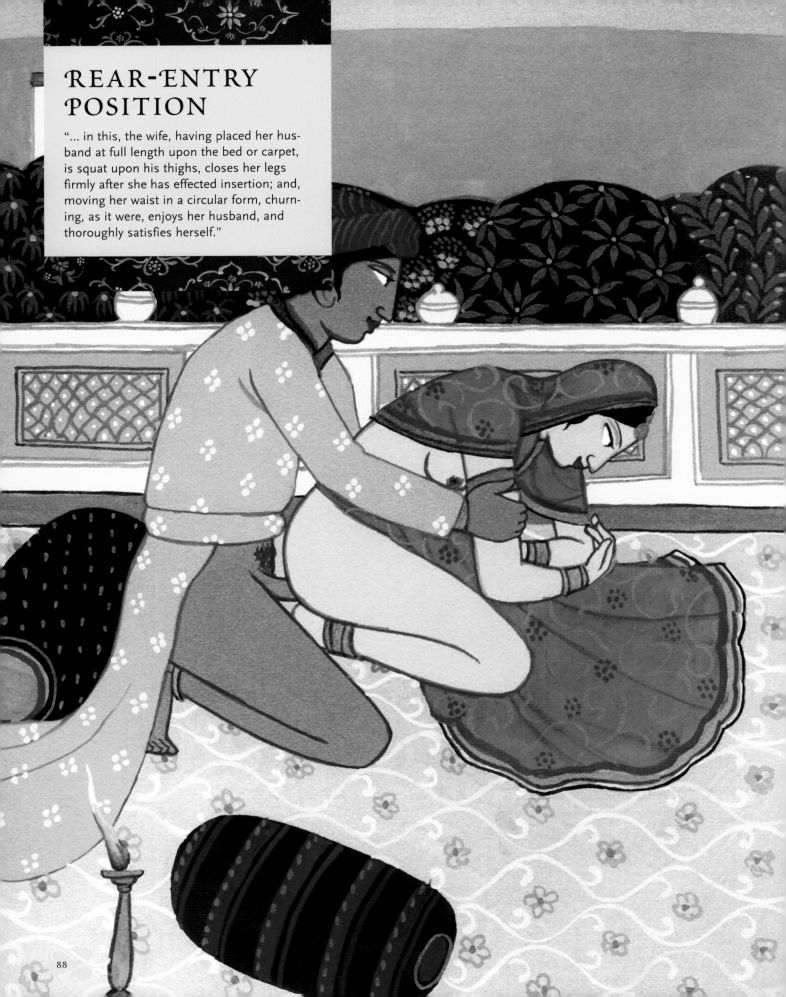

REAR-ENTRY POSITION

"... in this, the wife, having placed her husband at full length upon the bed or carpet, is squat upon his thighs, closes her legs firmly after she has effected insertion; and, moving her waist in a circular form, churning, as it were, enjoys her husband, and thoroughly satisfies herself."

The man lies on his back in this position, pulling his legs apart so his partner can sit between them. The woman, after penetration, balances herself on her hands and feet, "churning" and moving her body.

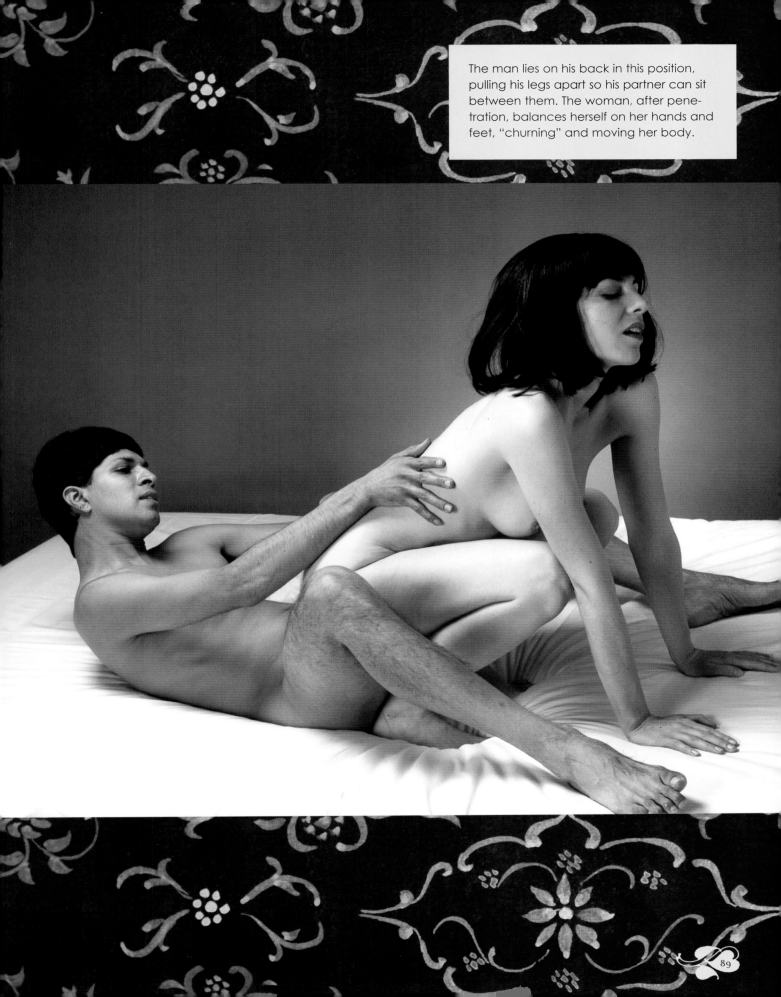

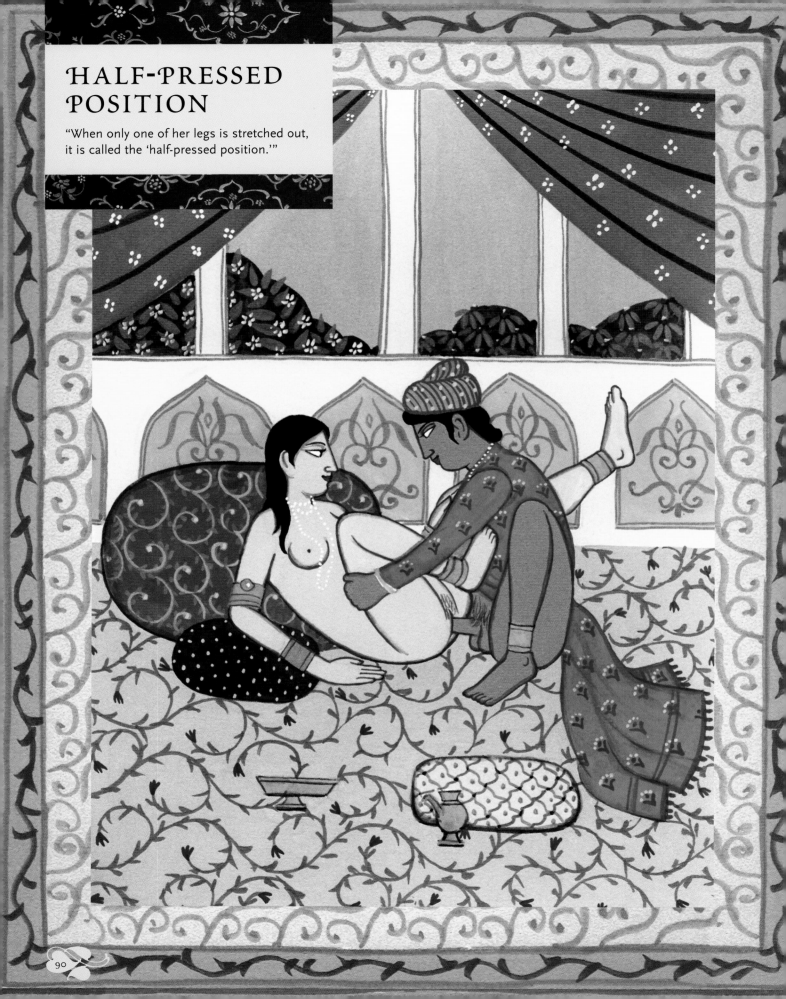

HALF-PRESSED
POSITION

"When only one of her legs is stretched out,
it is called the 'half-pressed position.'"

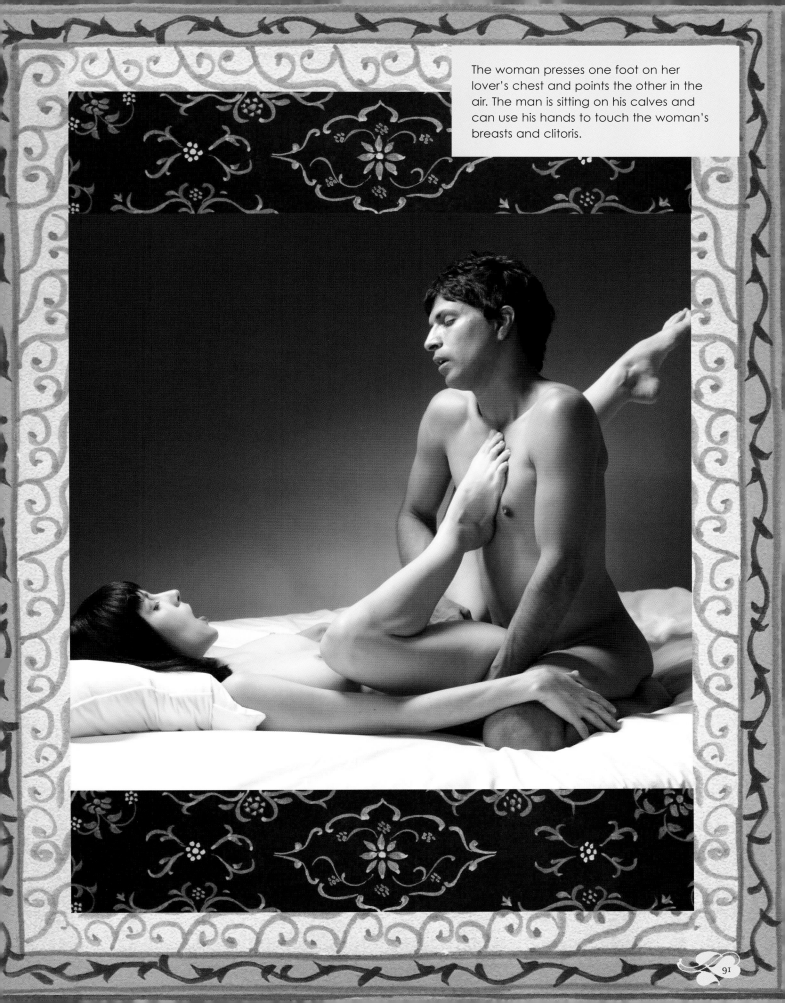

The woman presses one foot on her lover's chest and points the other in the air. The man is sitting on his calves and can use his hands to touch the woman's breasts and clitoris.

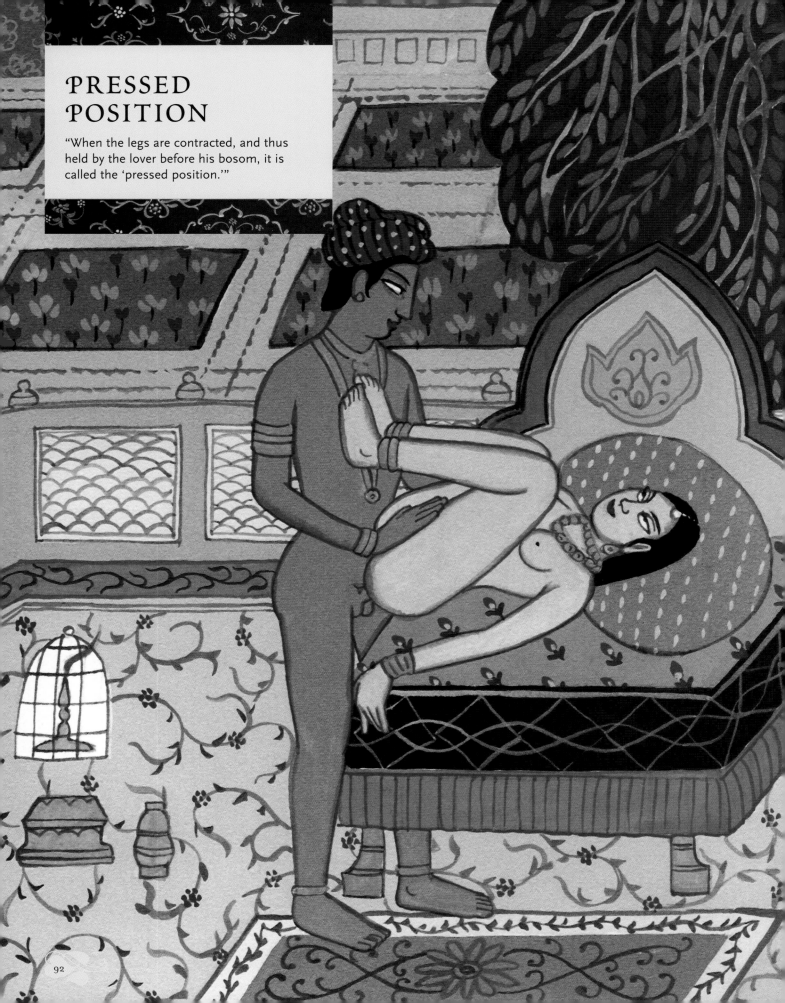

PRESSED
POSITION

"When the legs are contracted, and thus held by the lover before his bosom, it is called the 'pressed position.'"

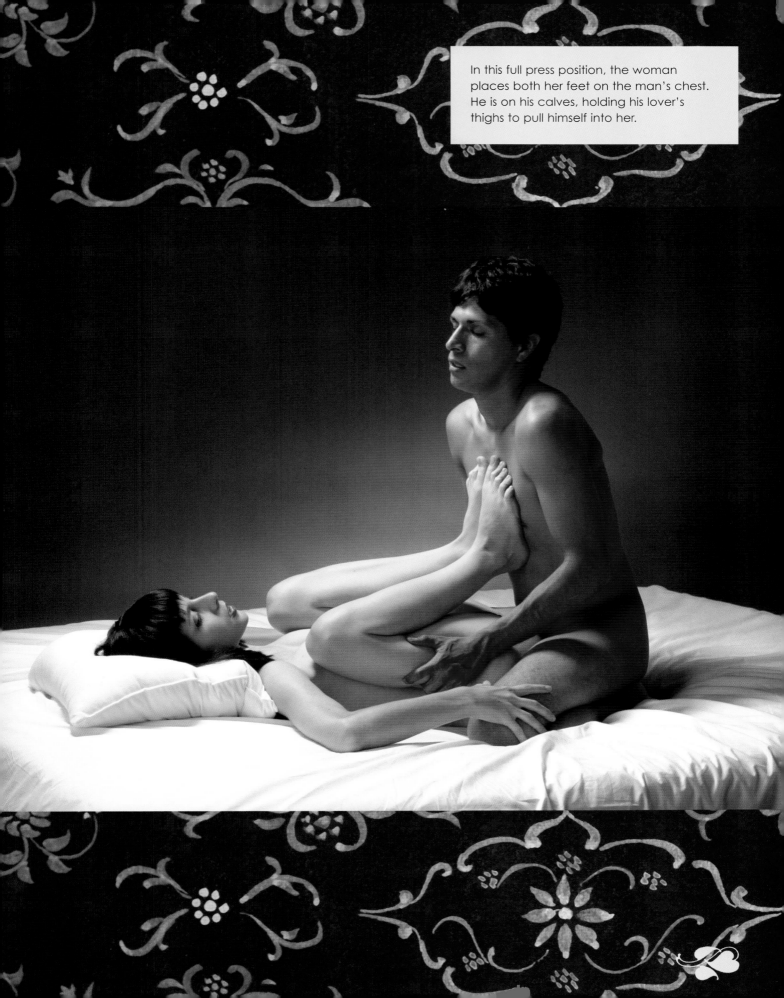

In this full press position, the woman places both her feet on the man's chest. He is on his calves, holding his lover's thighs to pull himself into her.

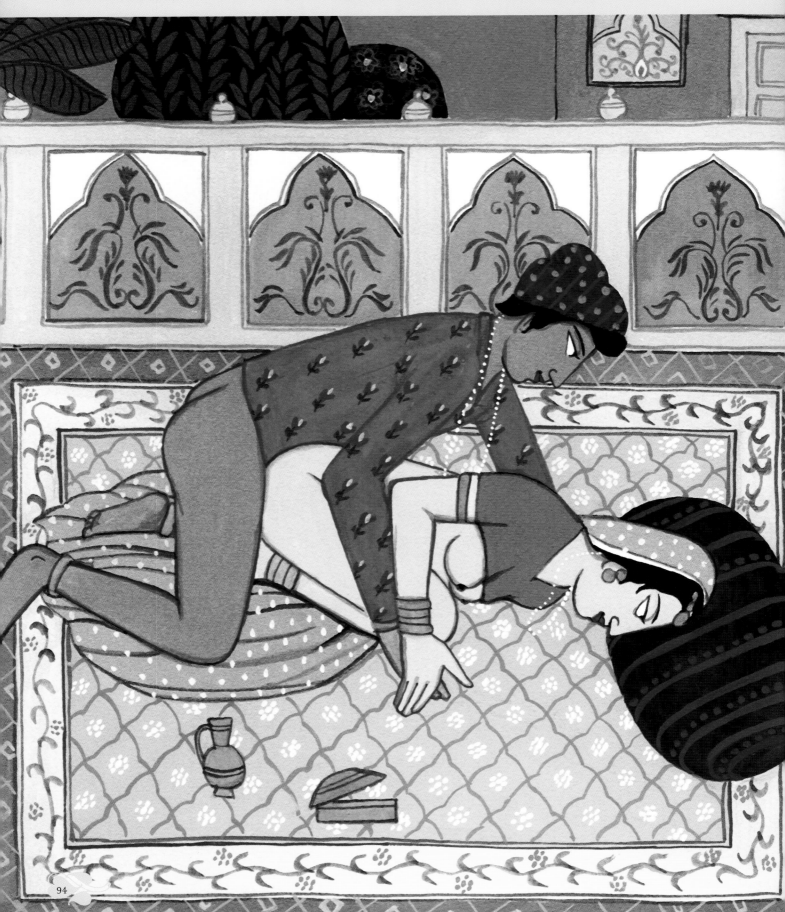

94

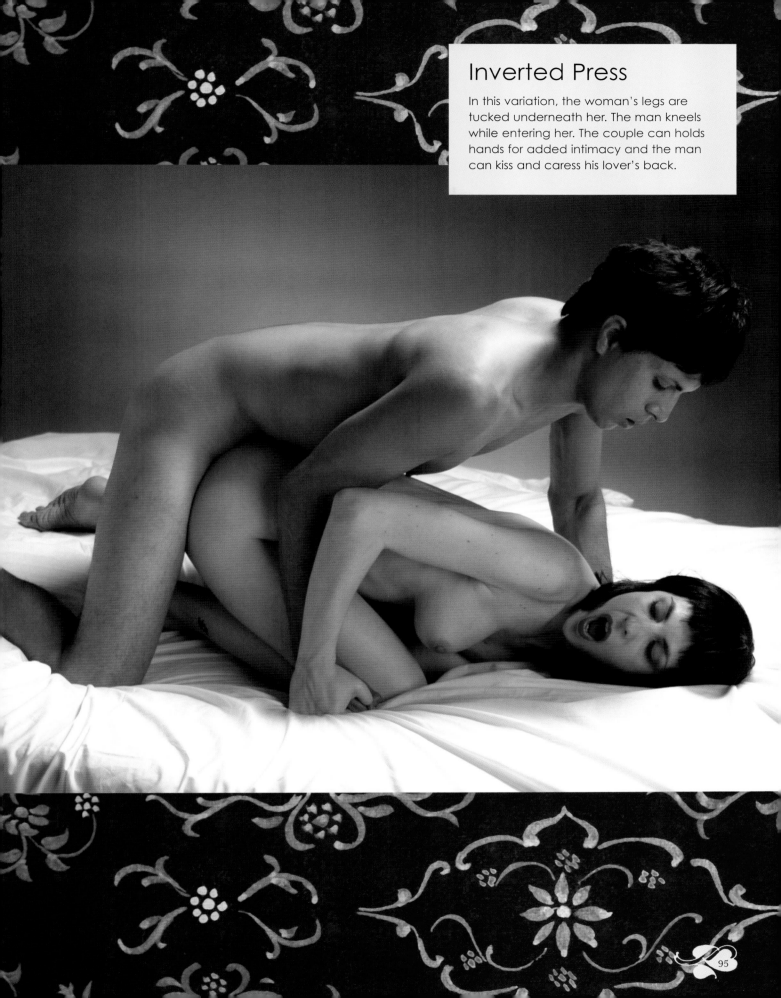

Inverted Press

In this variation, the woman's legs are tucked underneath her. The man kneels while entering her. The couple can holds hands for added intimacy and the man can kiss and caress his lover's back.

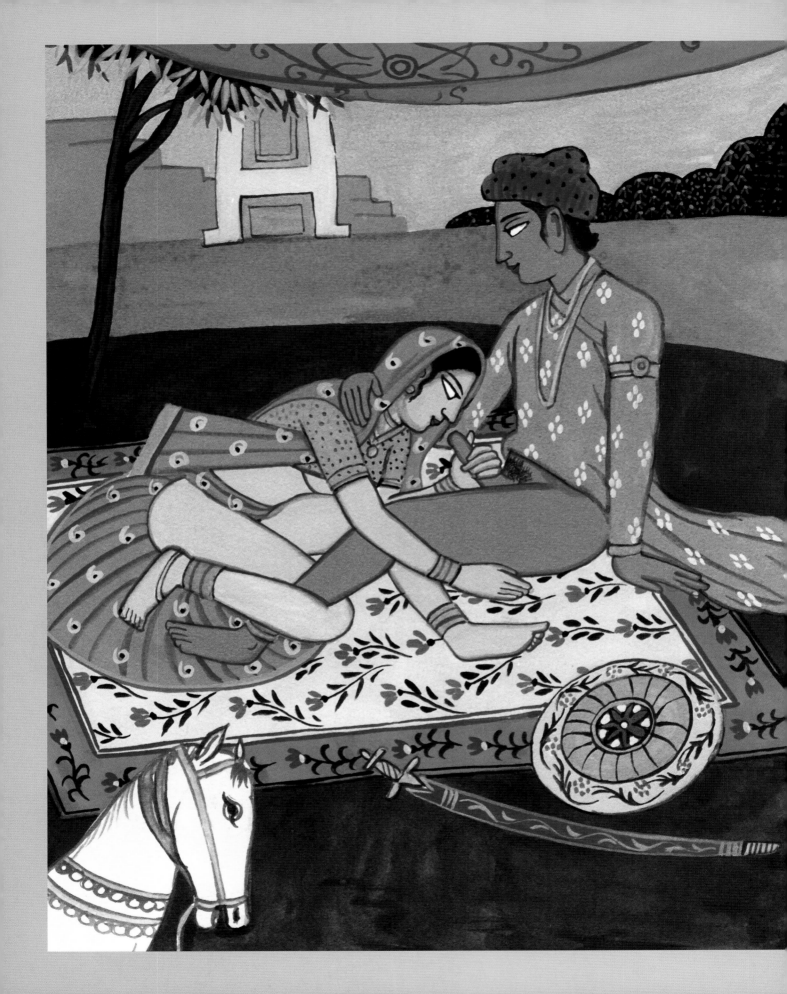

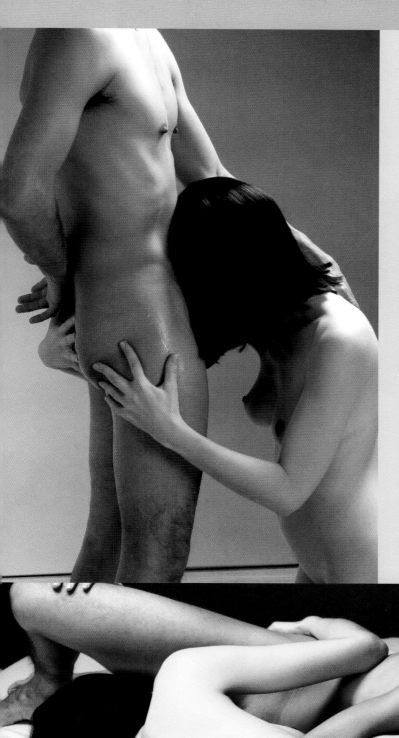

ORAL SEX

Vatsyayana dedicated an entire chapter to oral sex, as he knew the intrigue and raw pleasure that came with it. In addition to the male with female occurrences, within the *Kama Sutra* there are details of the frequency of male with male and female with female oral sex.

Vatsyayana divided male oral sex into eight stages, what begins with the woman simply kissing his penis, ends with her attempting to put his entire member into her mouth, and "swallowing up" its contents. The key to performing great oral sex, is communication. Ask what he or she likes/feels and dislikes. Sounds and facial expressions are also reliable indicators of what feels fabulous versus what is less effective. The *Kama Sutra* suggests that the giver start by kissing the penis, then proceed to licking and sucking. The intensity will vary with different partners. It is best not to discuss whether the woman should or should not swallow the semen.

Vatsyayana did not forget about the woman's pleasure. He suggests, "The way of doing this (i.e. of kissing the yoni) should be known from kissing the mouth." Instead of going directly for the clitoris, the man should first kiss her inner thighs and hips. Then, paying attention to what makes the woman moan with joy, he should use his tongue to give her as much pleasure—and as many orgasms— as he can.

In the *Kama Sutra* the Congress of a Crow position is what today is known as the "69 position." It says, "When a man and woman lie down in an inverted order, i.e. with the head of the one towards the feet of the other and carry on this congress, it is called the 'congress of a crow'" The couple should, at all times, pay attention to each other's needs in order to minimize discomfort and maximize pleasure.

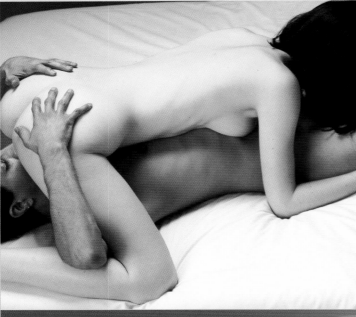

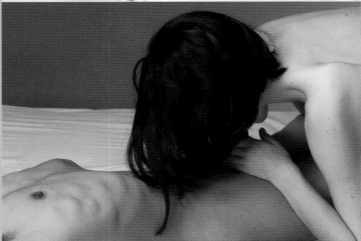

"THINGS REALLY GET STEAMY WHEN PARTNERS PLEASURE EACH OTHER AT THE SAME TIME."

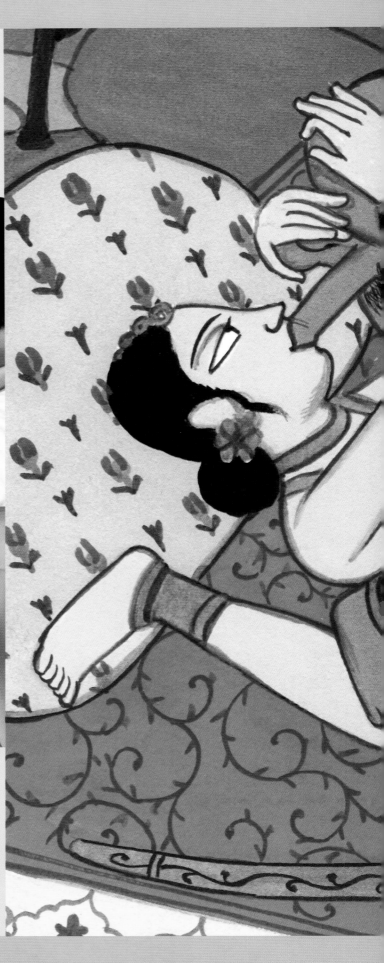

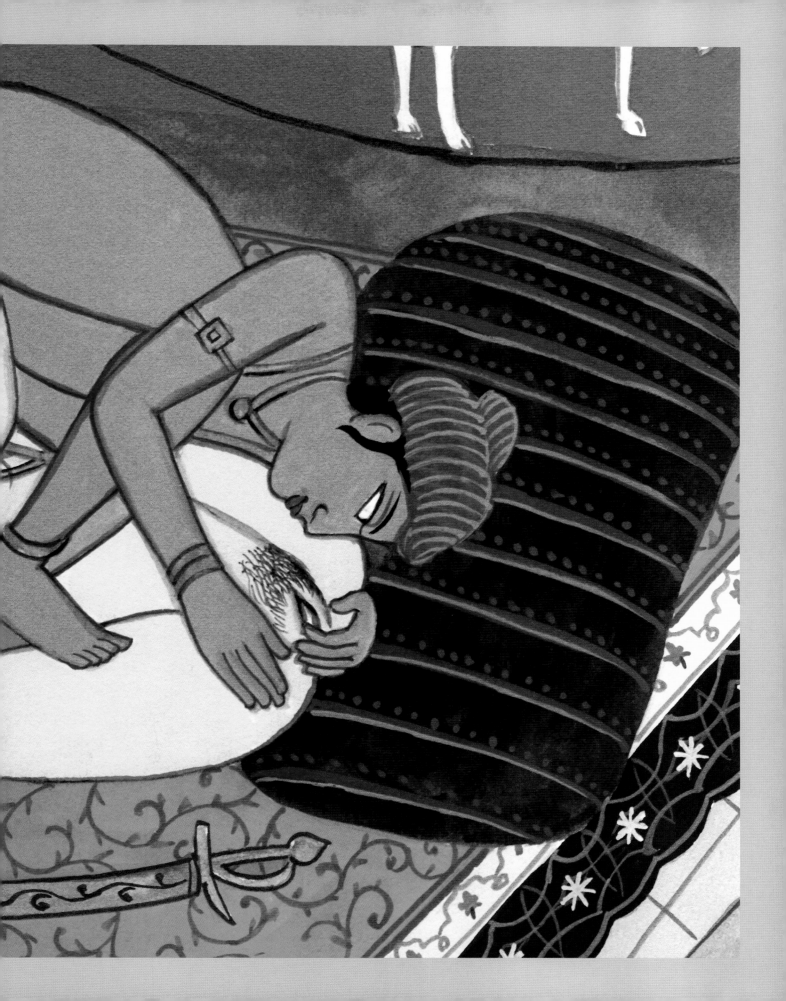

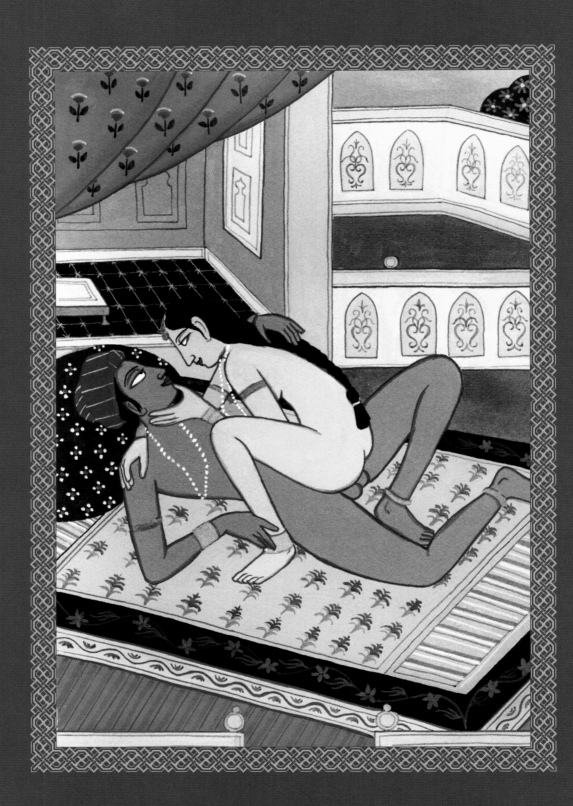

5 TOP POSITIONS

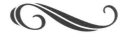

A woman's pleasure was always a key issue in the Kama Sutra. Vatsyayana told men—as they were the book's intended audience—how to pleasure her, and what "the signs of the enjoyment and satisfaction of the woman" are. He also encouraged men to allow the woman to do the "work" sometimes, meaning she should be on top of him. In the Top Positions, the woman is in control and uses her body to bring pleasure to both her and her partner.

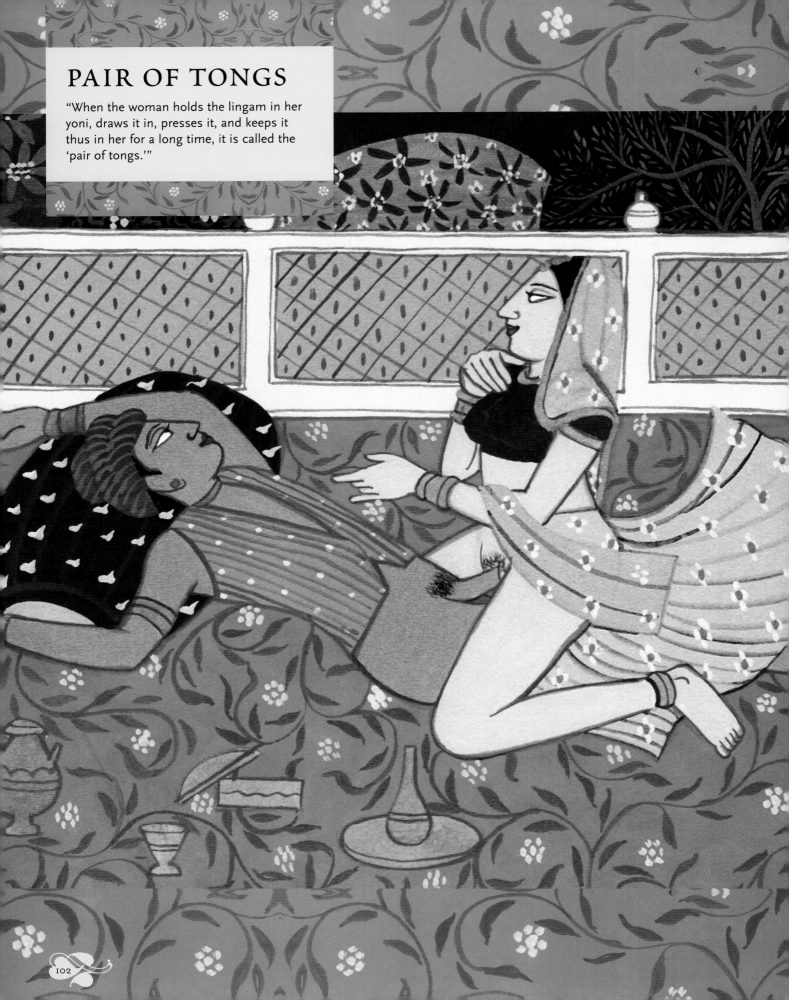

PAIR OF TONGS

"When the woman holds the lingam in her yoni, draws it in, presses it, and keeps it thus in her for a long time, it is called the 'pair of tongs.'"

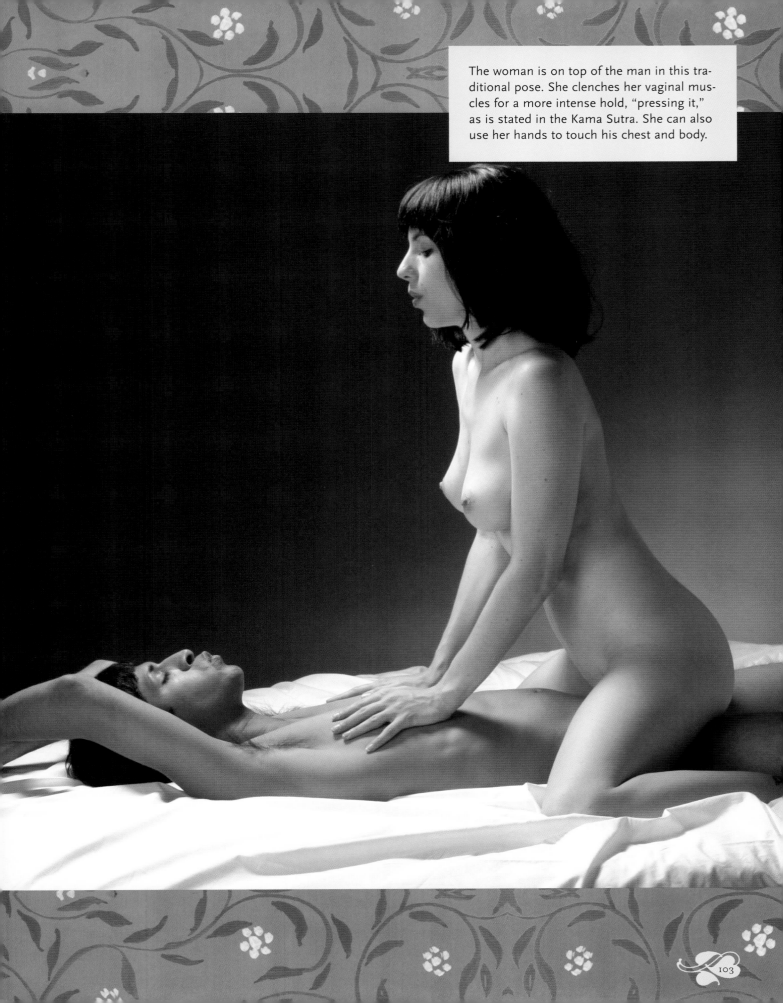

The woman is on top of the man in this traditional pose. She clenches her vaginal muscles for a more intense hold, "pressing it," as is stated in the Kama Sutra. She can also use her hands to touch his chest and body.

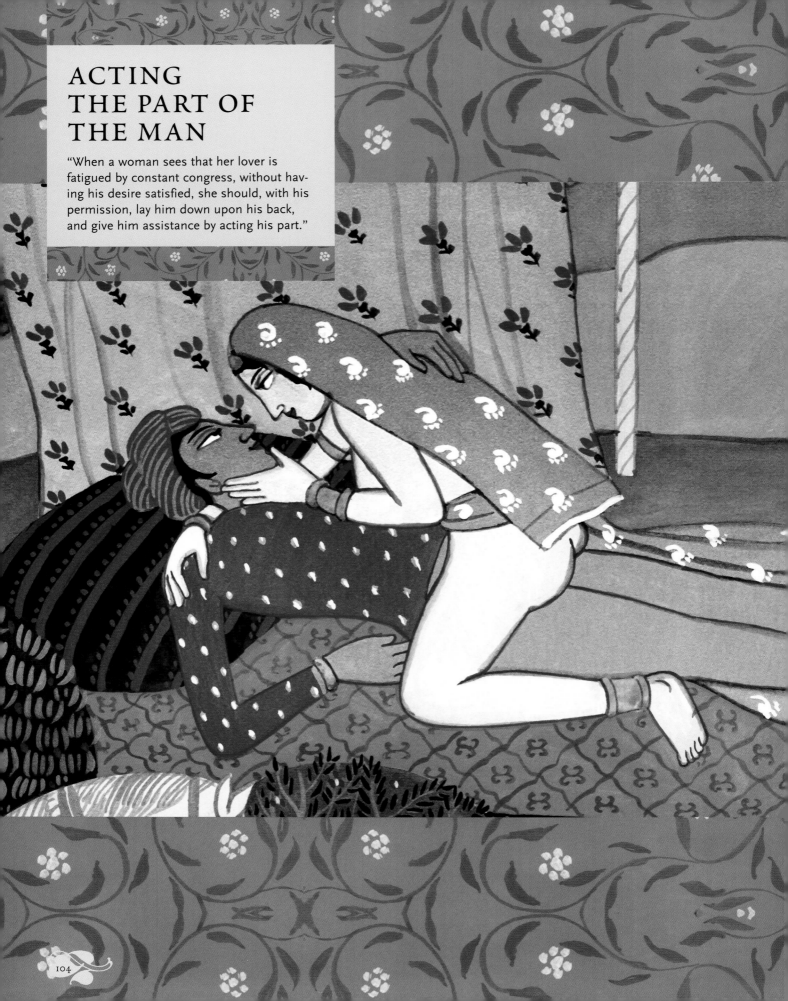

ACTING THE PART OF THE MAN

"When a woman sees that her lover is fatigued by constant congress, without having his desire satisfied, she should, with his permission, lay him down upon his back, and give him assistance by acting his part."

The man lies on his back in this position, as the woman acts "his part." She controls the pace, and both enjoy a great deal of pleasure.

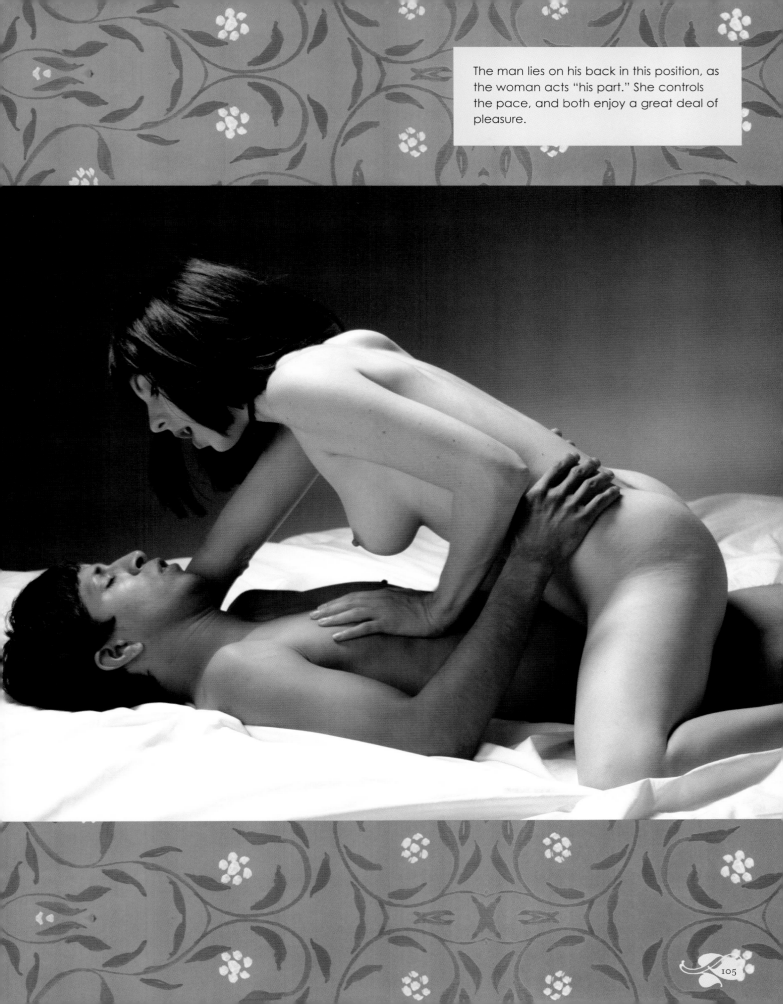

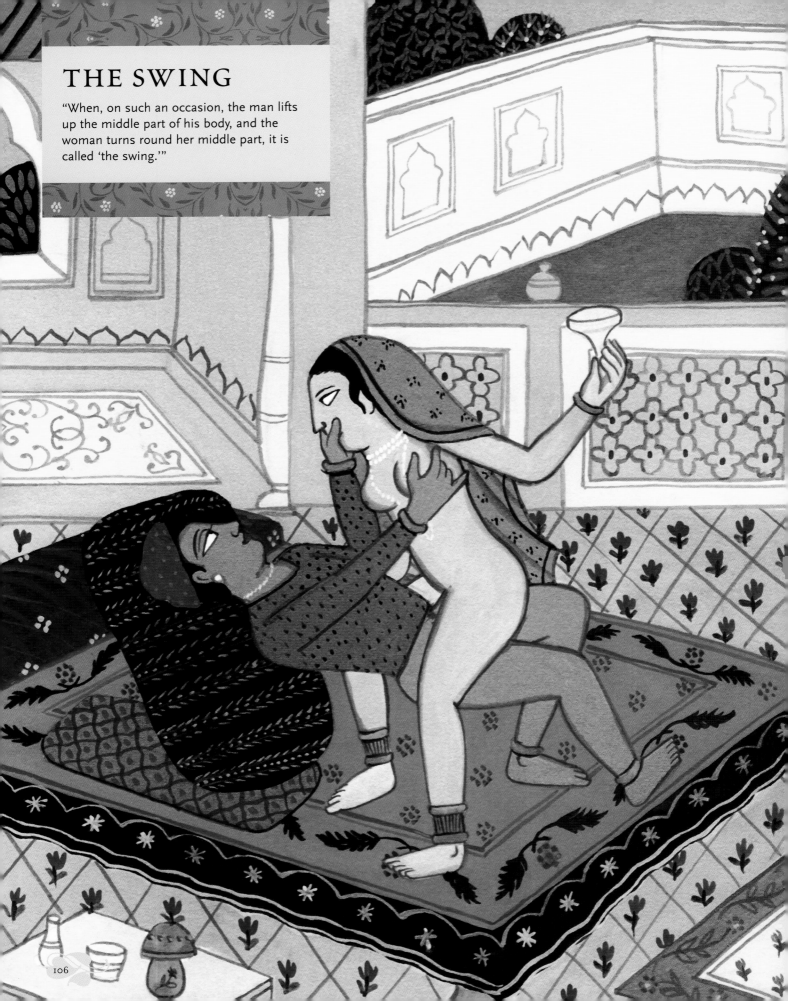

THE SWING

"When, on such an occasion, the man lifts up the middle part of his body, and the woman turns round her middle part, it is called 'the swing.'"

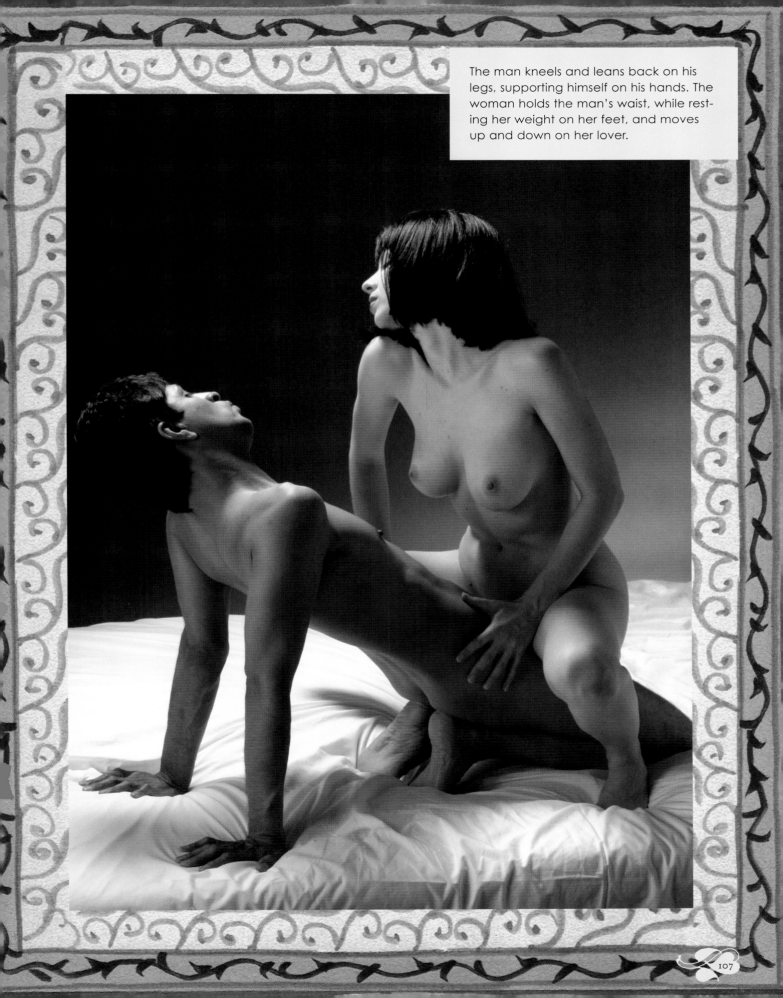

The man kneels and leans back on his legs, supporting himself on his hands. The woman holds the man's waist, while resting her weight on her feet, and moves up and down on her lover.

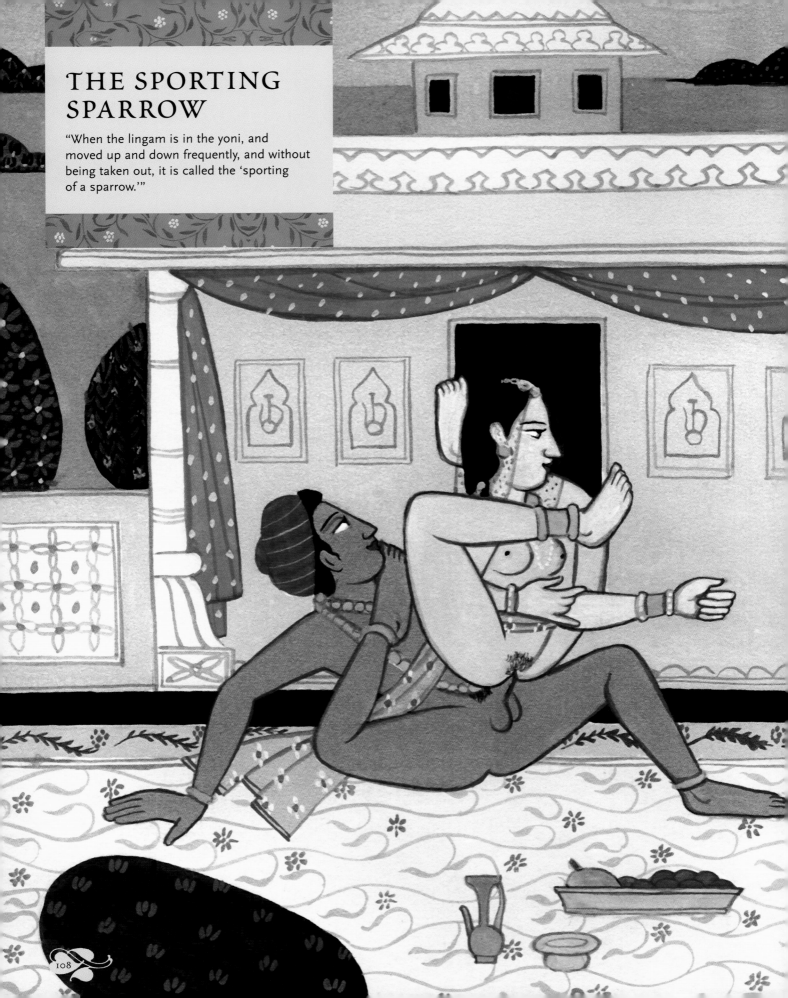

THE SPORTING SPARROW

"When the lingam is in the yoni, and moved up and down frequently, and without being taken out, it is called the 'sporting of a sparrow.'"

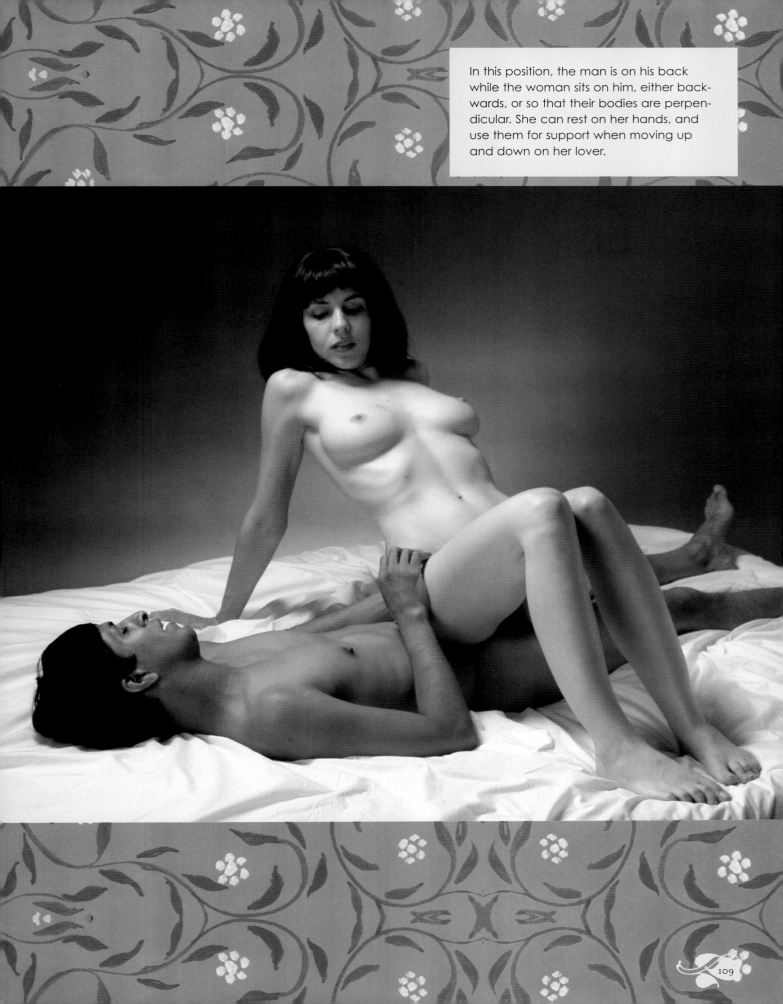

In this position, the man is on his back while the woman sits on him, either backwards, or so that their bodies are perpendicular. She can rest on her hands, and use them for support when moving up and down on her lover.

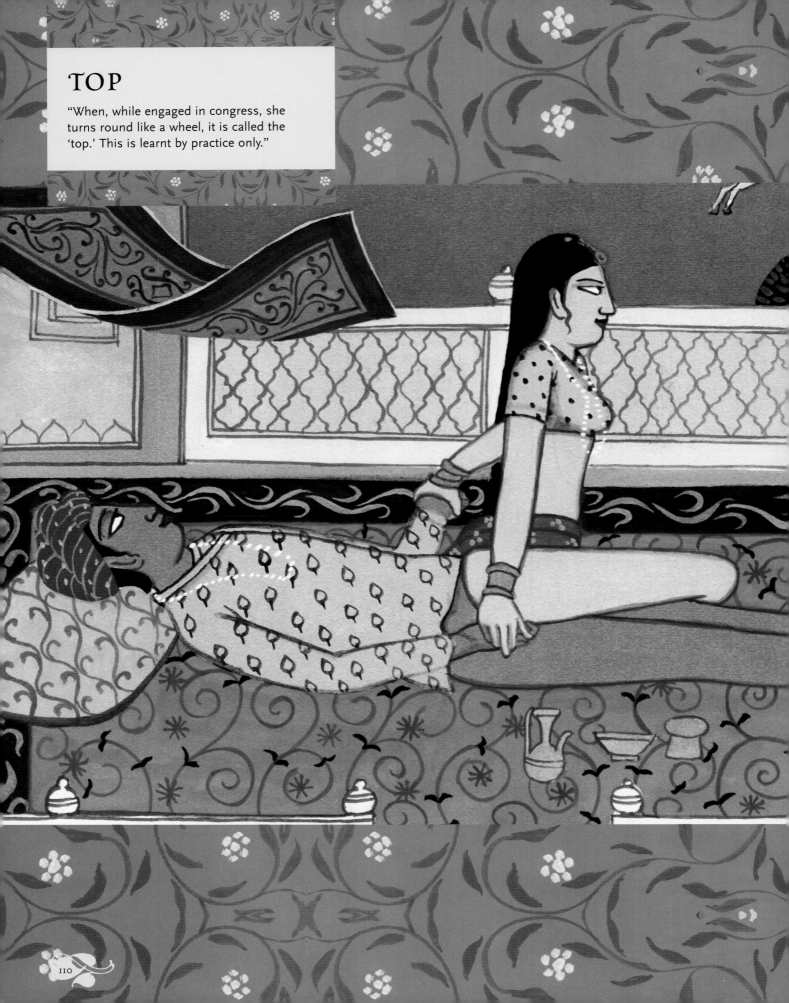

TOP

"When, while engaged in congress, she turns round like a wheel, it is called the 'top.' This is learnt by practice only."

This position is similar to the Turning Position, except the woman is on top, instead of the man. She sits on her lover and rotates her body, appreciating the different angles of penetration that each point offers. Both partners stay steady and relaxed.

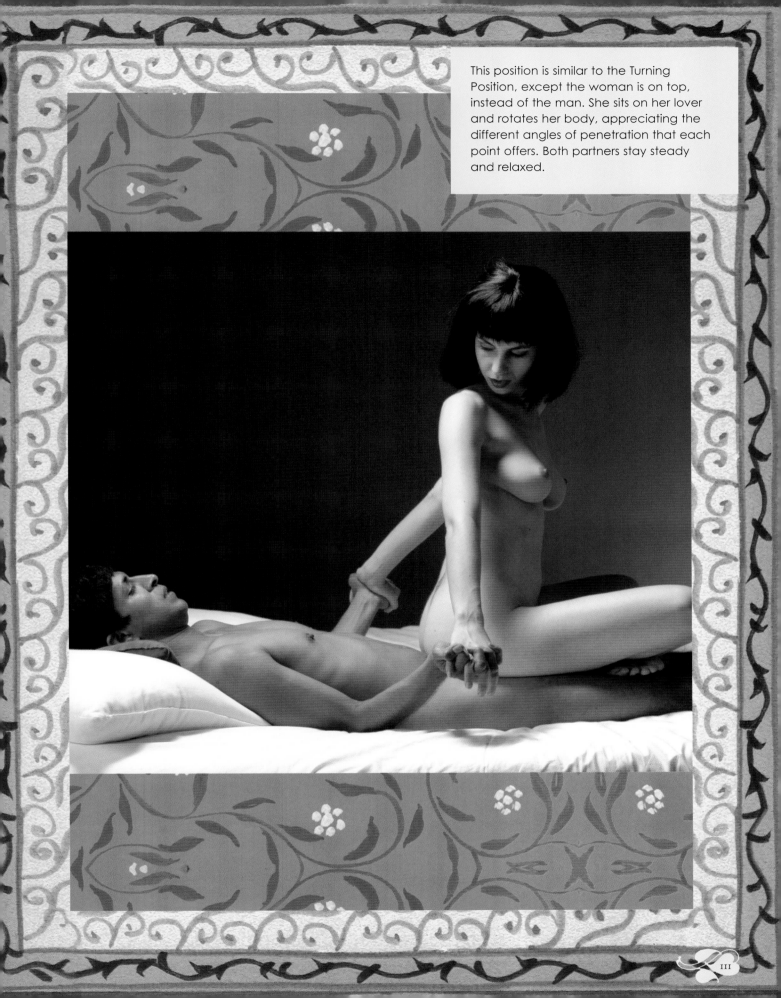

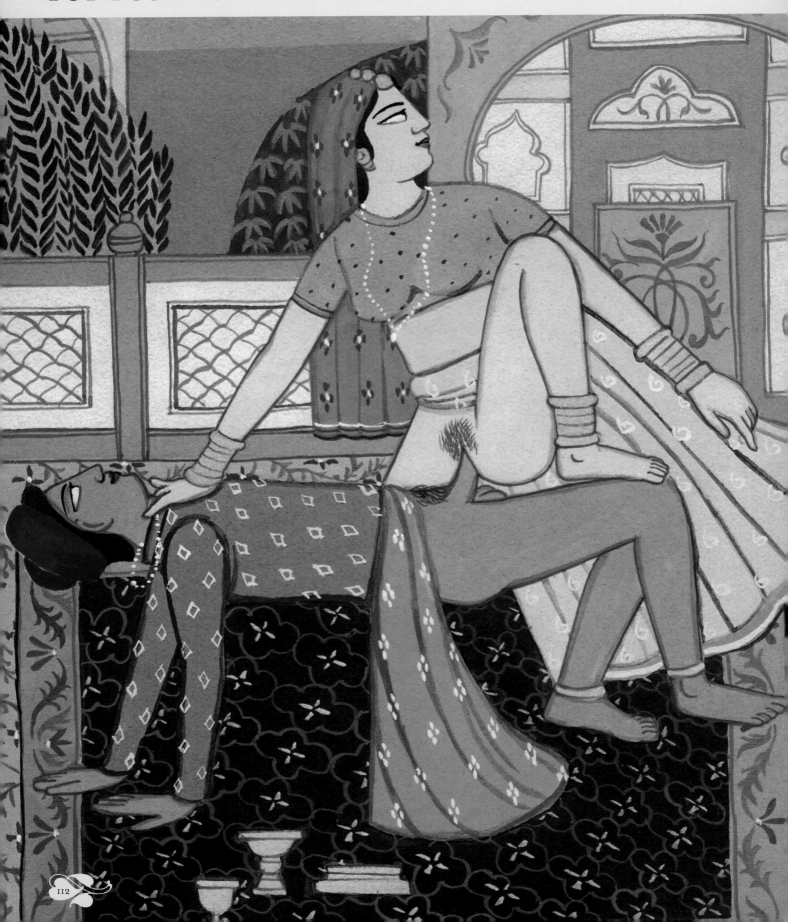

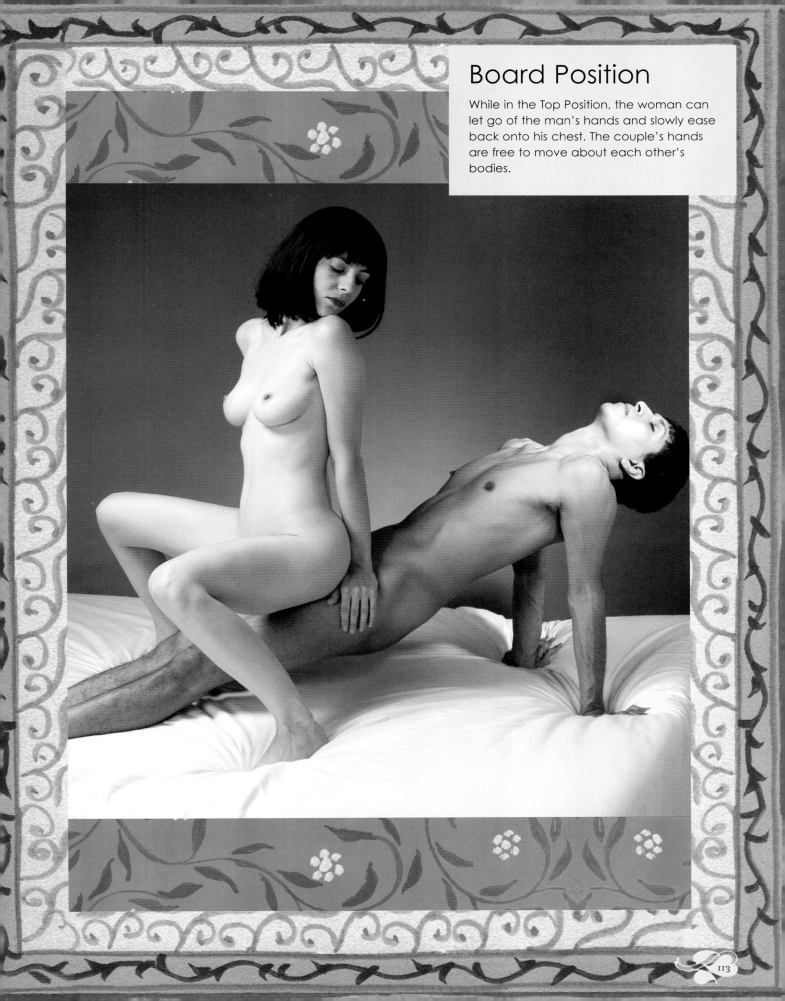

Board Position

While in the Top Position, the woman can let go of the man's hands and slowly ease back onto his chest. The couple's hands are free to move about each other's bodies.

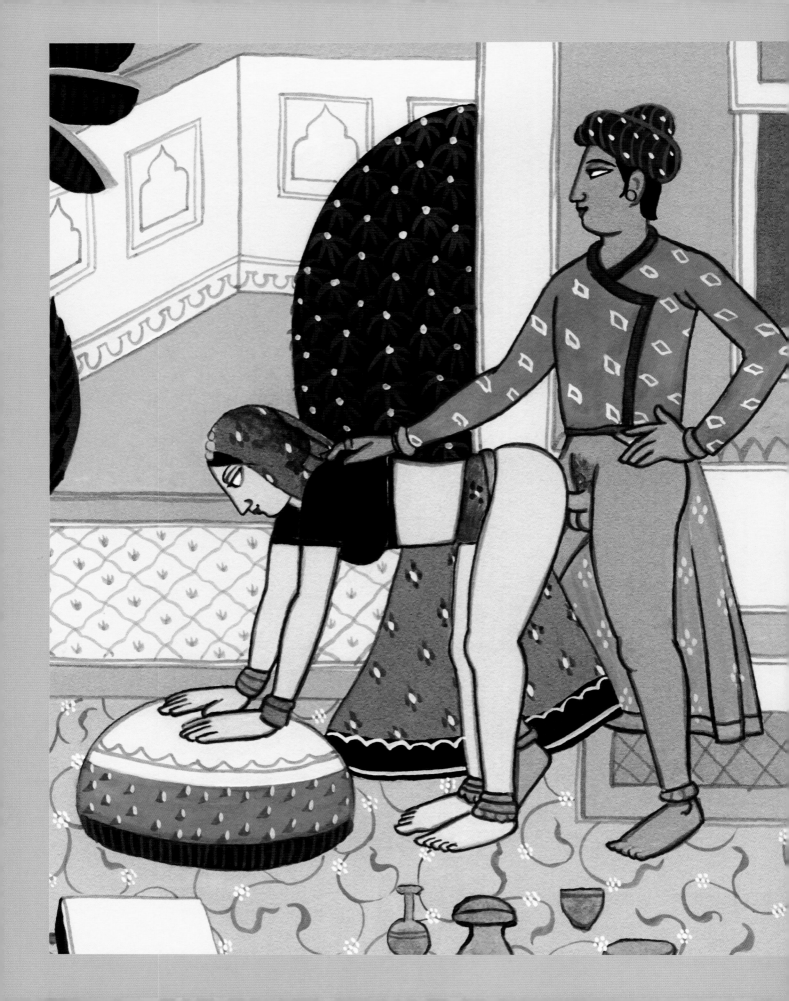

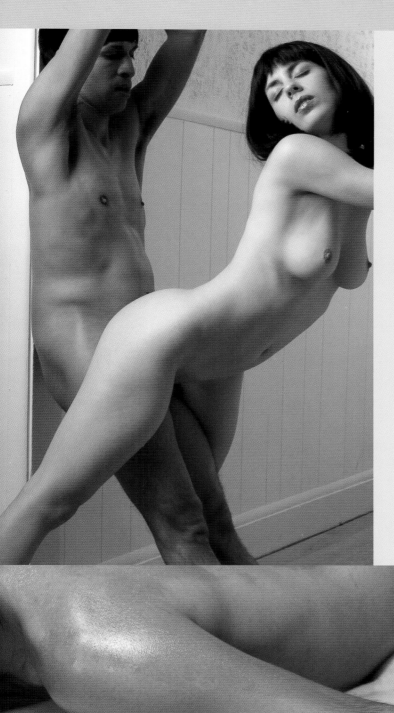

INTIMACY

While sex in and of itself can be an amazing, fulfilling, mind-blowing experience, what can take it to an even higher plane is the intimacy shared—in a look or touch. It could be a spontaneous meeting of minds and bodies or stepping back to take a new look at a longtime companion, somebody you would feel comfortable doing things with that you couldn't do with a stranger.

So, how do you get more intimate with your lover? Let it evolve, have fun, break out of your routine—tie him up; blindfold her. By increasing abandon and letting down your guard, you will automatically begin to trust each other and increase your level of intimacy as well as working the kinks out of (and into) your sex play.

Light some candles, caress every inch of your lover's body, and if you are too shy to say what it is you want in bed, take a sheet of paper and write your desires down, then fold it 7 times or until you cannot fold it any longer, and present it to your lover as a present.

Understand the importance of a trusting relationship. It is written in the *Kama Sutra* that, "... in the same manner a loving pair become blind with passion in the heat of congress, and go on with great impetuosity, paying not the least regard to excess." And if trust is already established between the two of you, there are everyday things that can increase the intimacy of a relationship.

Communication is imperative, not only about sex, but about life in general. Feeling committed to and accepted by your partner will automatically kick intimacy up a notch. Speak freely about bedroom likes and dislikes, as well as life goals, aspirations, and dreams. Without even realizing it, you will have laid the foundation for great sex and a lasting intimacy that will burn on much longer than any candle.

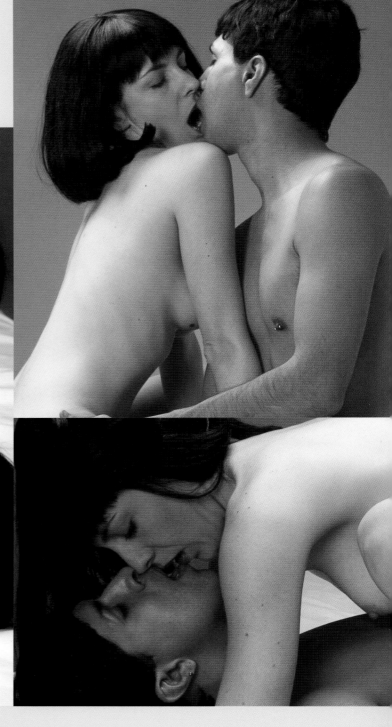

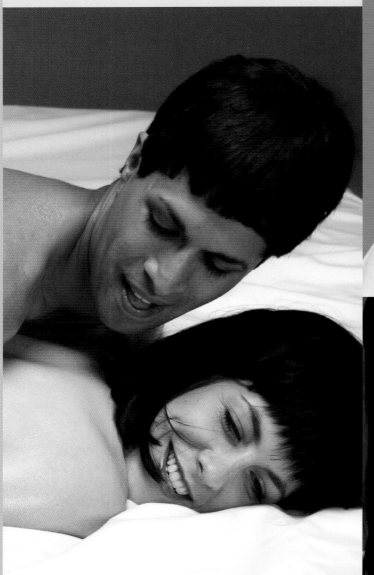

"SPEAK FREELY ABOUT BEDROOM LIKES AND DISLIKES, AS WELL AS LIFE GOALS, ASPIRATIONS, AND DREAMS."

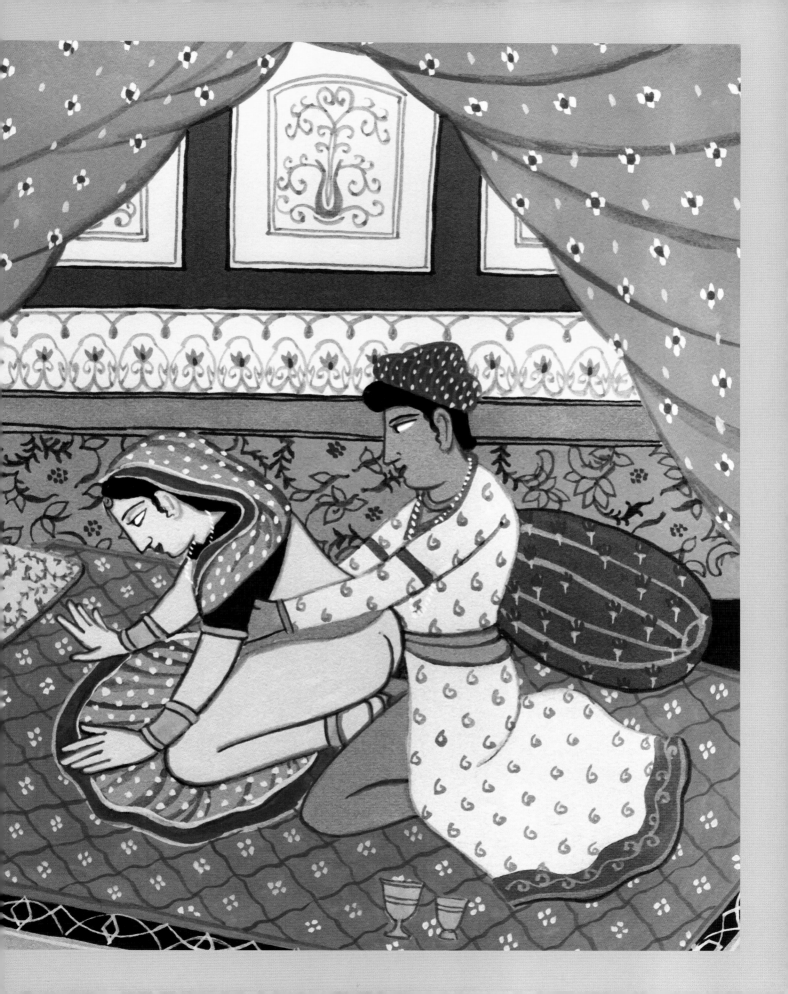

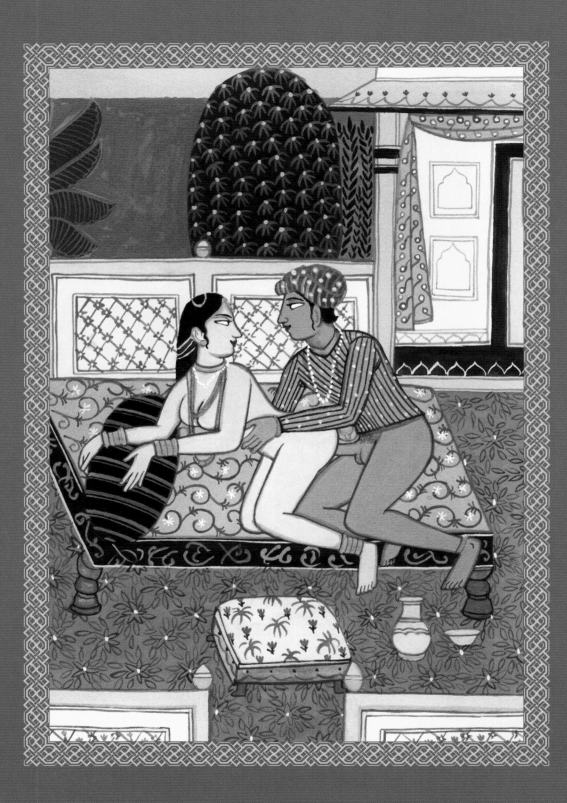

ANIMAL POSITIONS

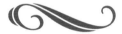

Vatsyayana encouraged readers to imitate the lovemaking techniques of the animals. In these positions, the woman should make sure she is always comfortable, and the man should always embrace and caress her body. She should reciprocate, to make the overall experience more fulfilling.

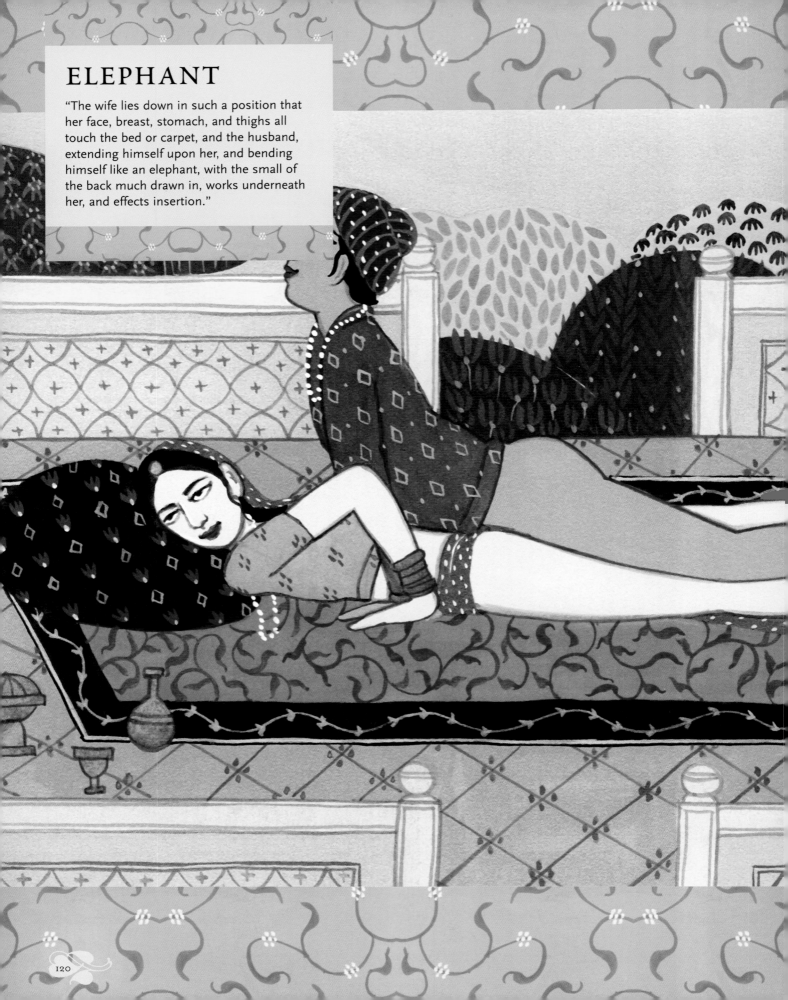

ELEPHANT

"The wife lies down in such a position that her face, breast, stomach, and thighs all touch the bed or carpet, and the husband, extending himself upon her, and bending himself like an elephant, with the small of the back much drawn in, works underneath her, and effects insertion."

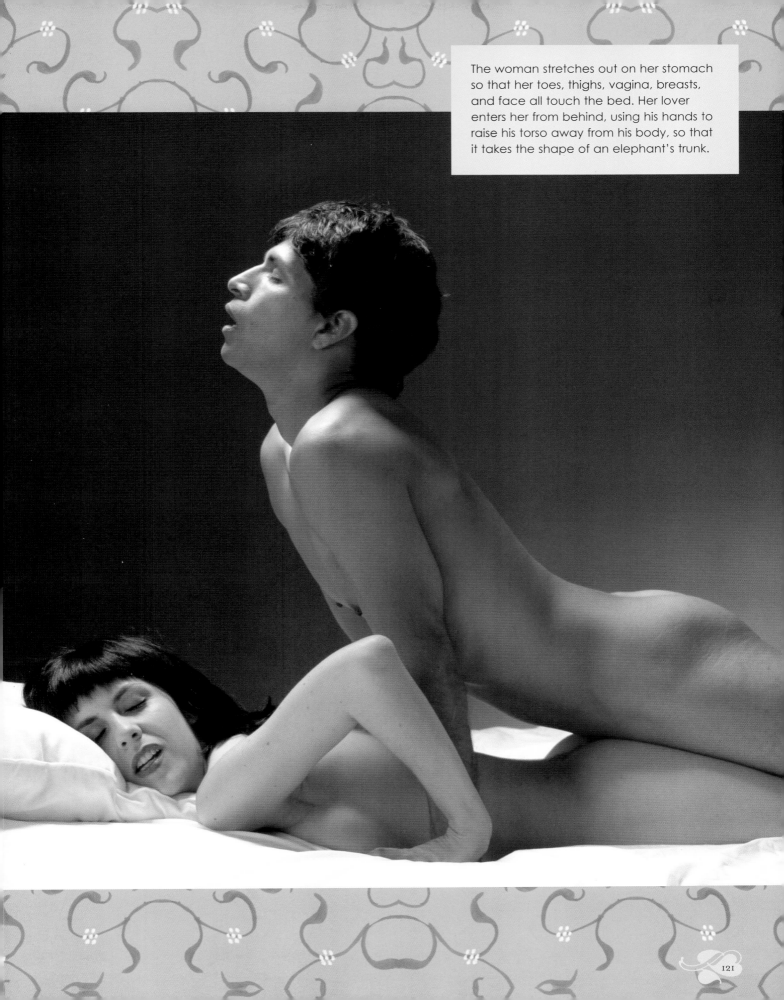

The woman stretches out on her stomach so that her toes, thighs, vagina, breasts, and face all touch the bed. Her lover enters her from behind, using his hands to raise his torso away from his body, so that it takes the shape of an elephant's trunk.

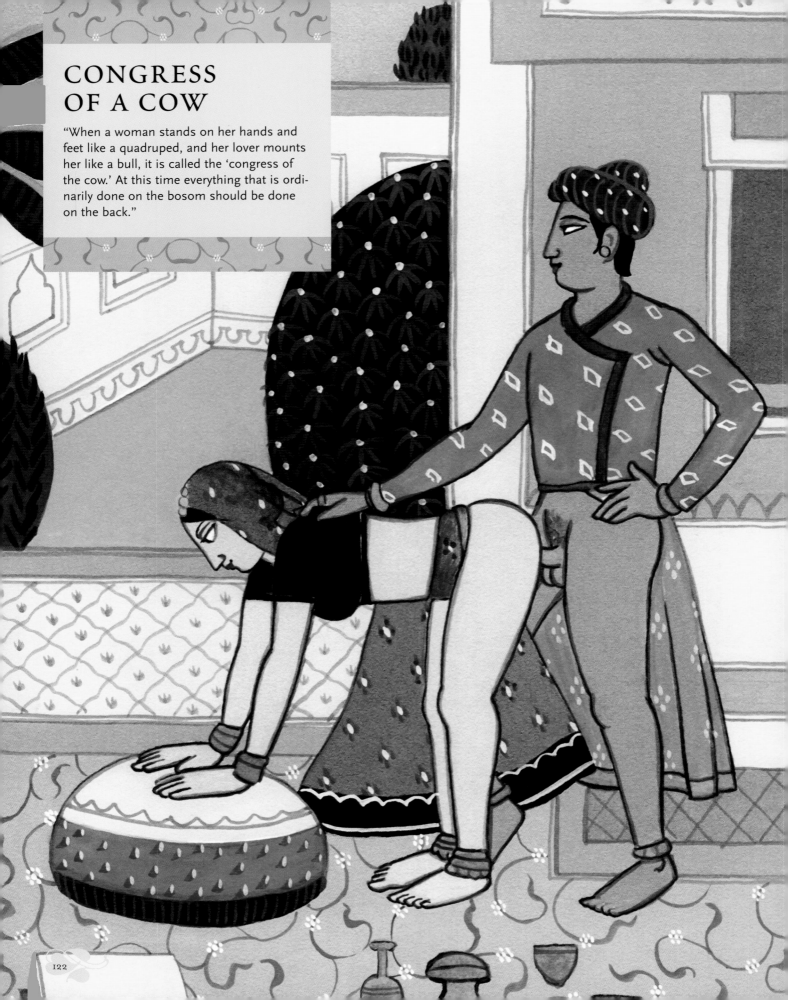

CONGRESS
OF A COW

"When a woman stands on her hands and feet like a quadruped, and her lover mounts her like a bull, it is called the 'congress of the cow.' At this time everything that is ordinarily done on the bosom should be done on the back."

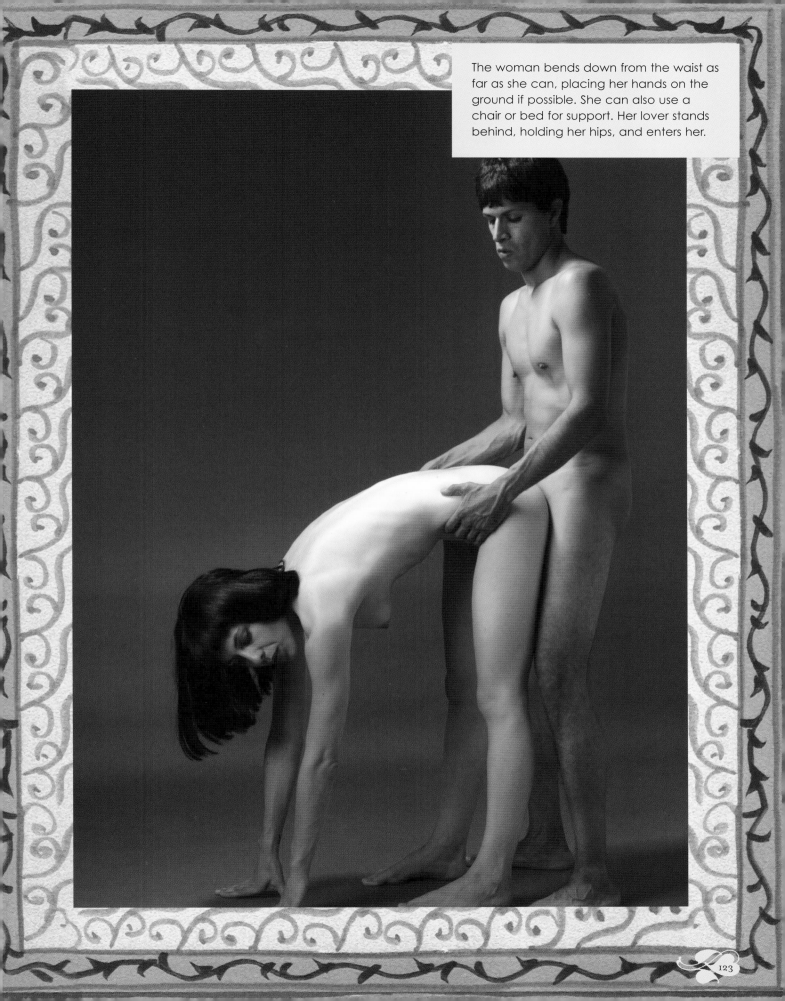

The woman bends down from the waist as far as she can, placing her hands on the ground if possible. She can also use a chair or bed for support. Her lover stands behind, holding her hips, and enters her.

123

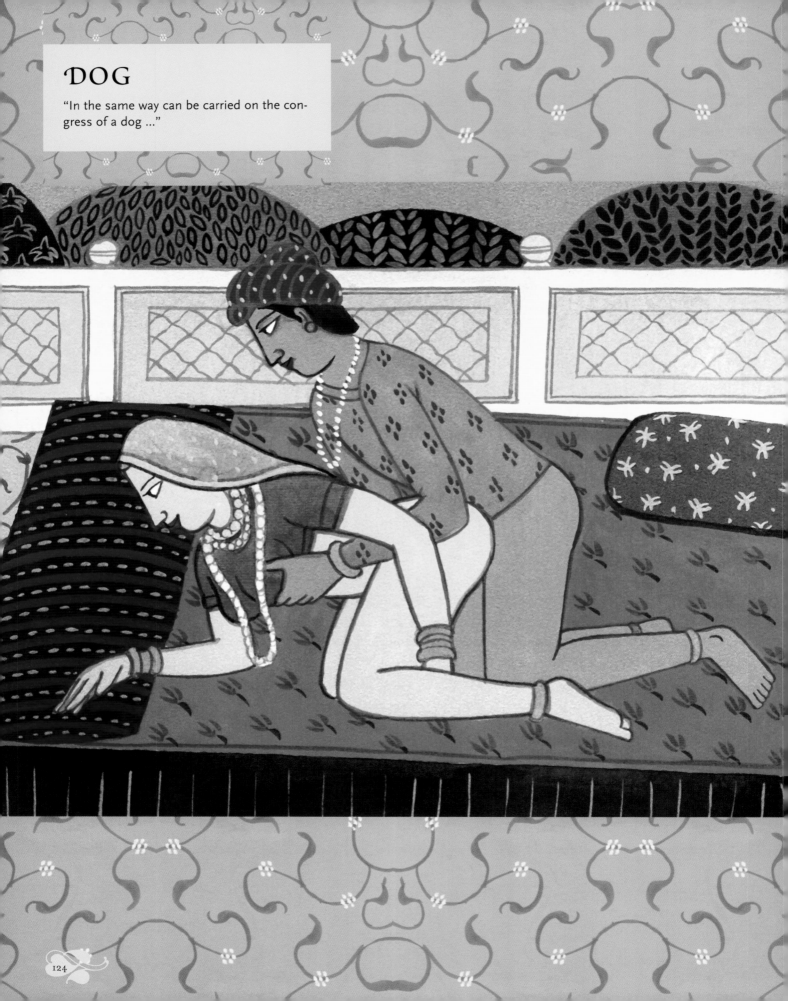

DOG

"In the same way can be carried on the congress of a dog ..."

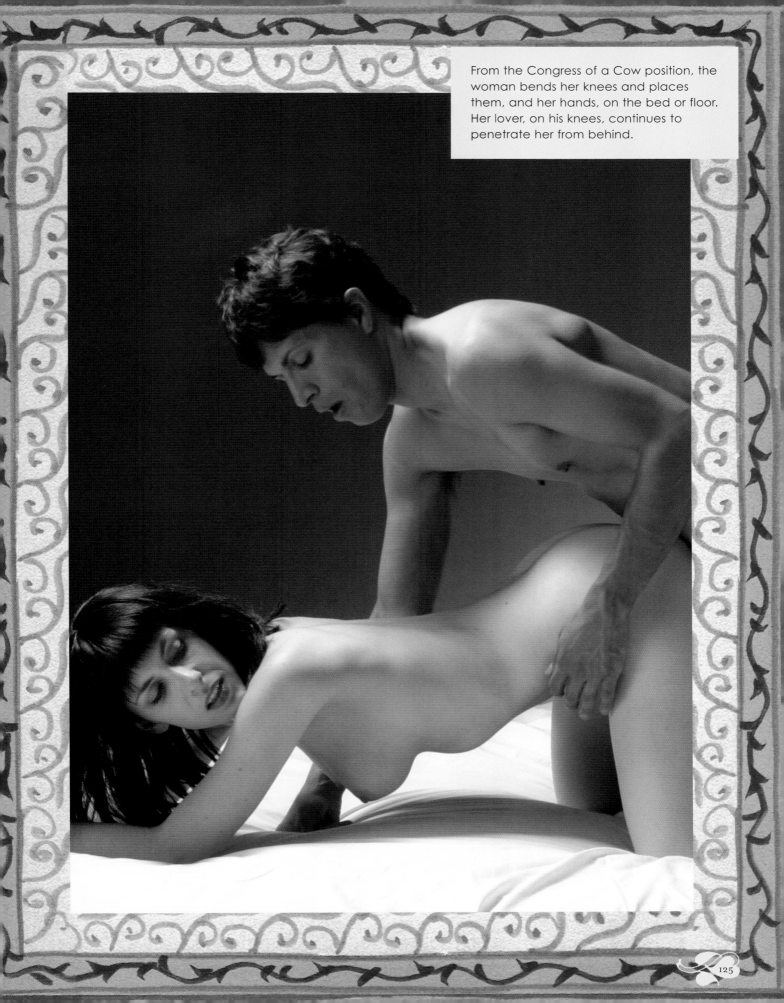

From the Congress of a Cow position, the woman bends her knees and places them, and her hands, on the bed or floor. Her lover, on his knees, continues to penetrate her from behind.

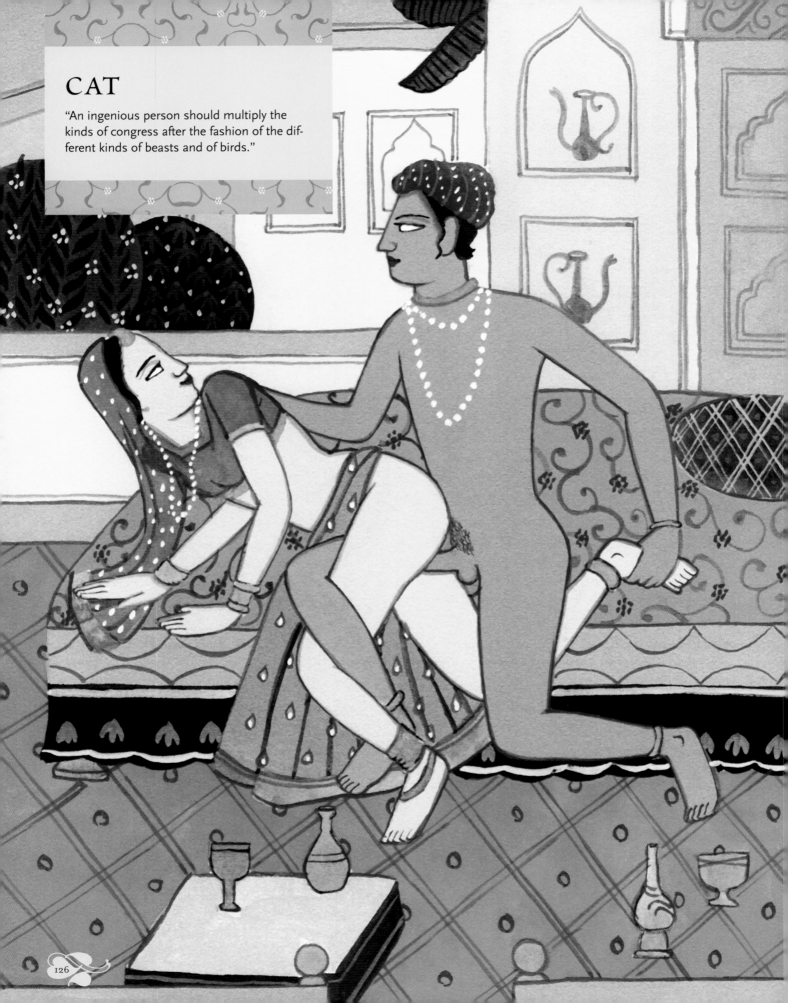

CAT

"An ingenious person should multiply the kinds of congress after the fashion of the different kinds of beasts and of birds."

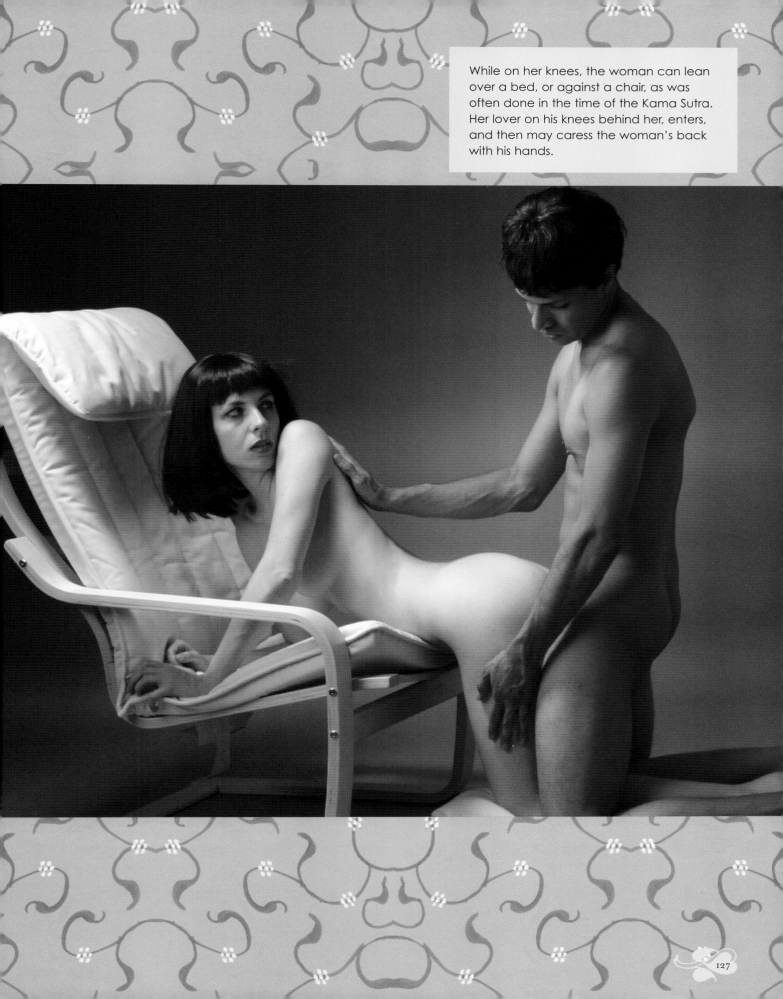

While on her knees, the woman can lean over a bed, or against a chair, as was often done in the time of the Kama Sutra. Her lover on his knees behind her, enters, and then may caress the woman's back with his hands.

127

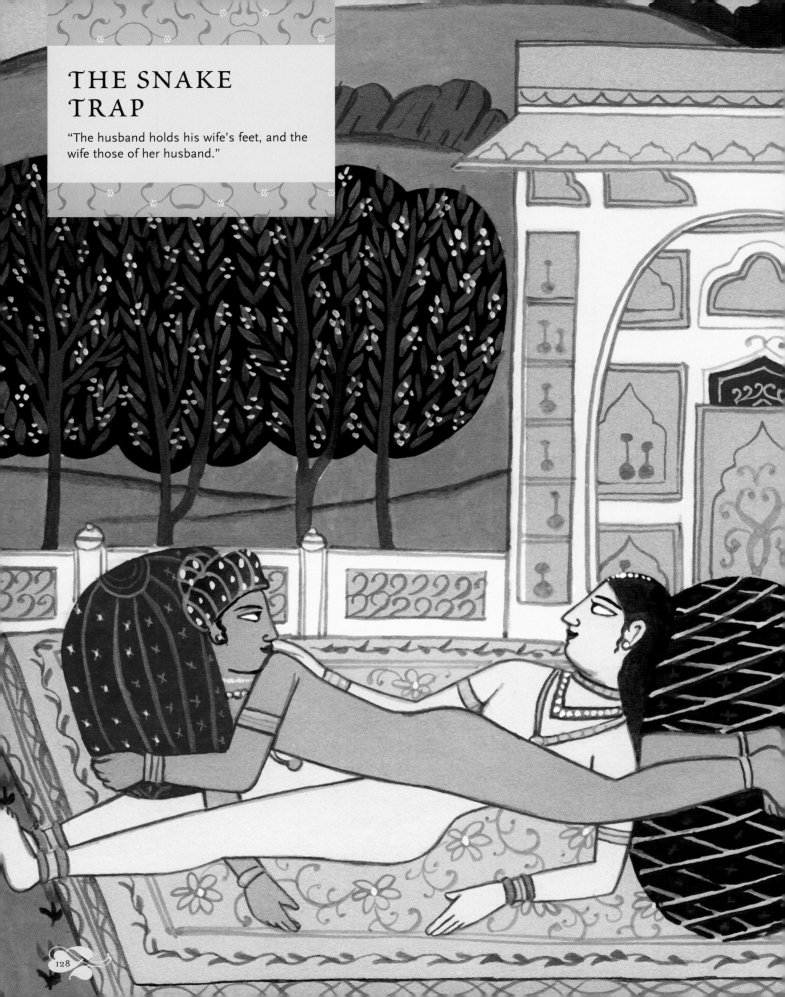

THE SNAKE TRAP

"The husband holds his wife's feet, and the wife those of her husband."

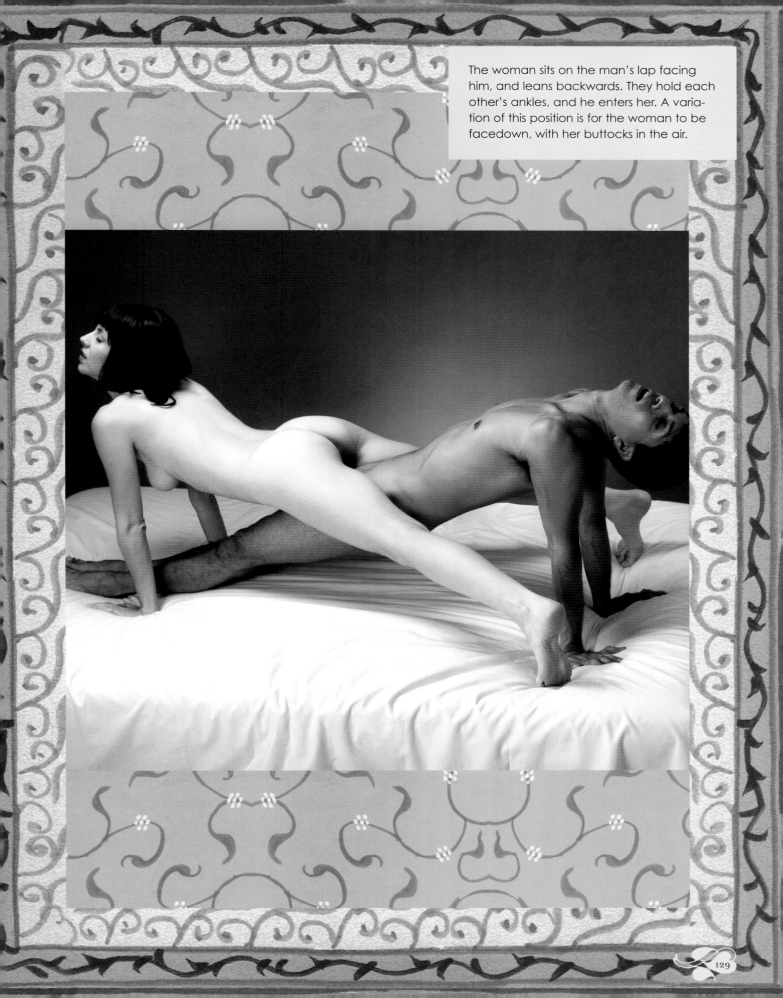

The woman sits on the man's lap facing
him, and leans backwards. They hold each
other's ankles, and he enters her. A variation of this position is for the woman to be
facedown, with her buttocks in the air.

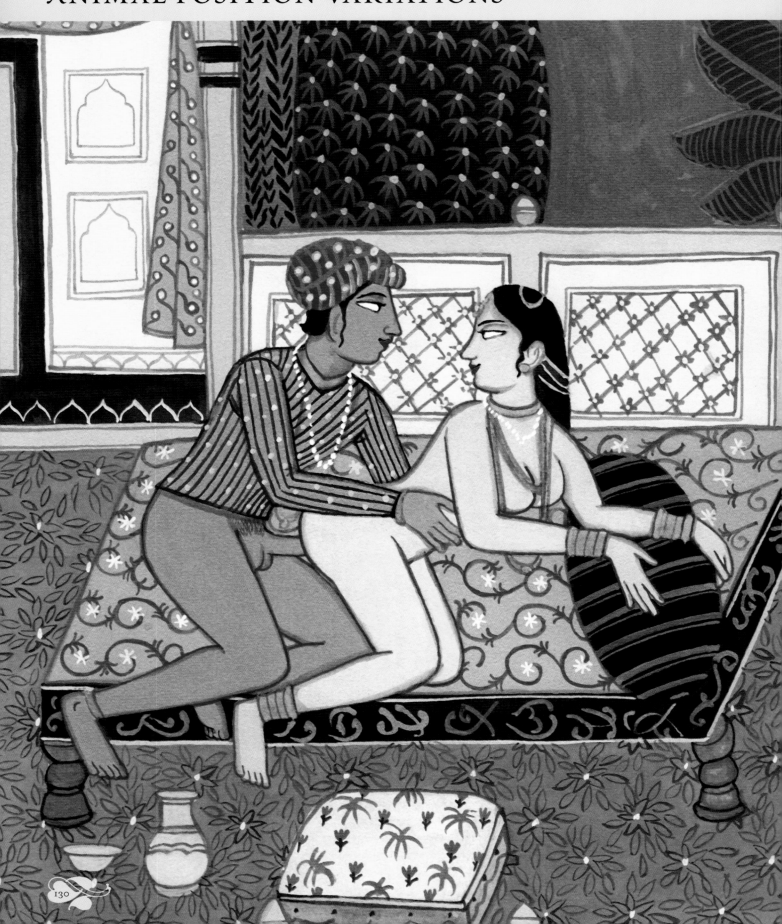

Tiger Position

In this variation of the Cat position, the woman stretches one of her legs out and bends the other against her lover. He continues to penetrate her from behind.

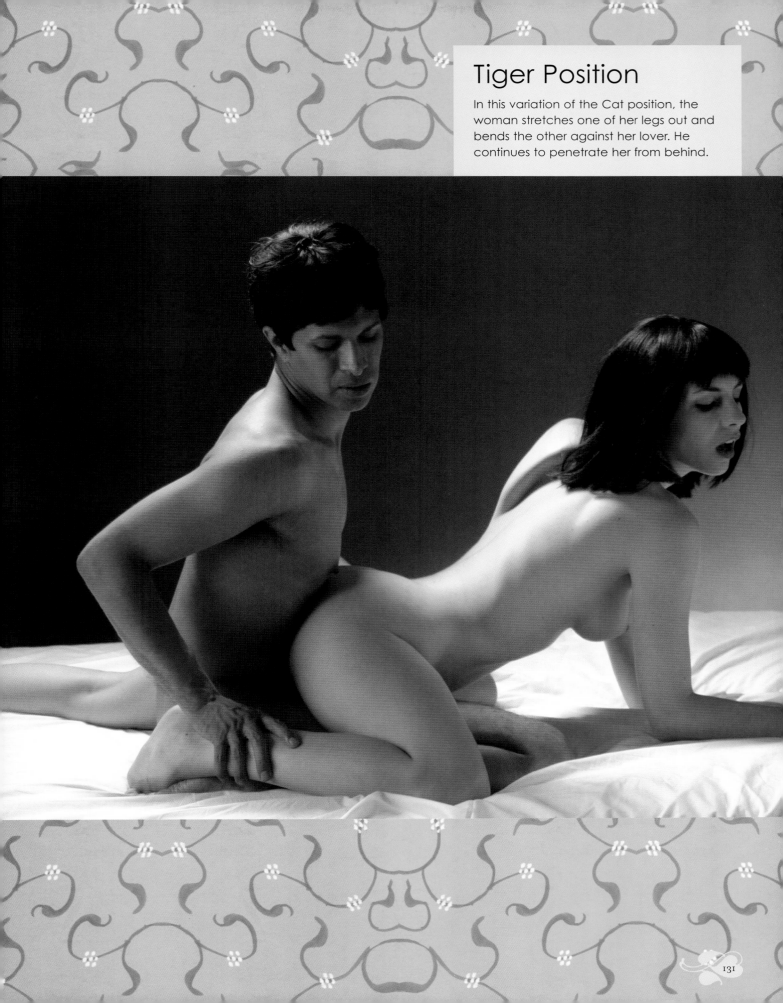

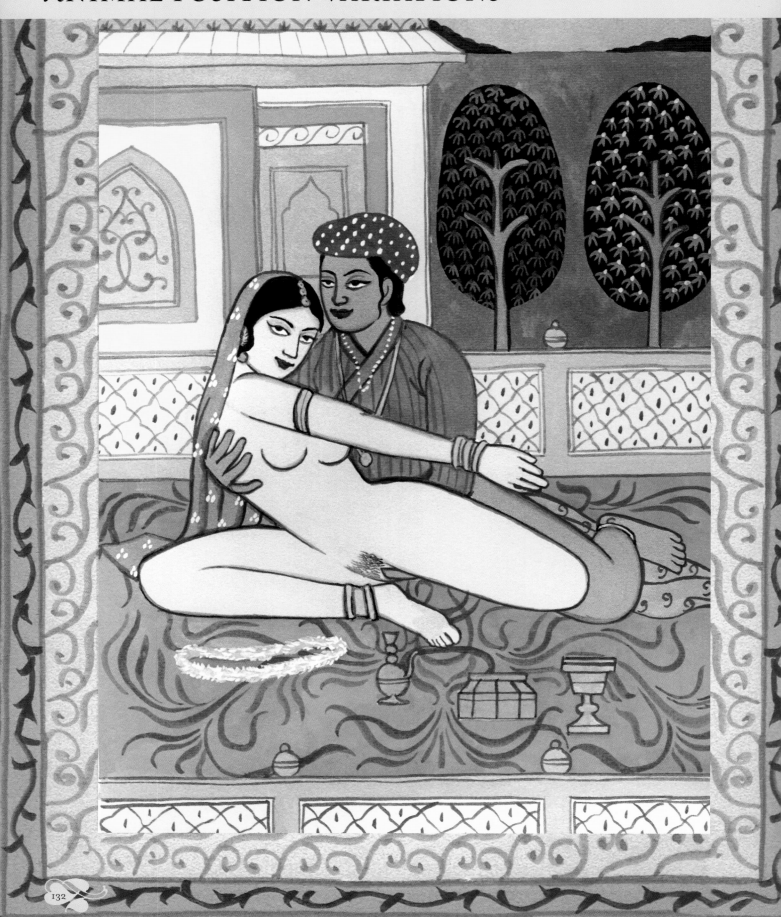

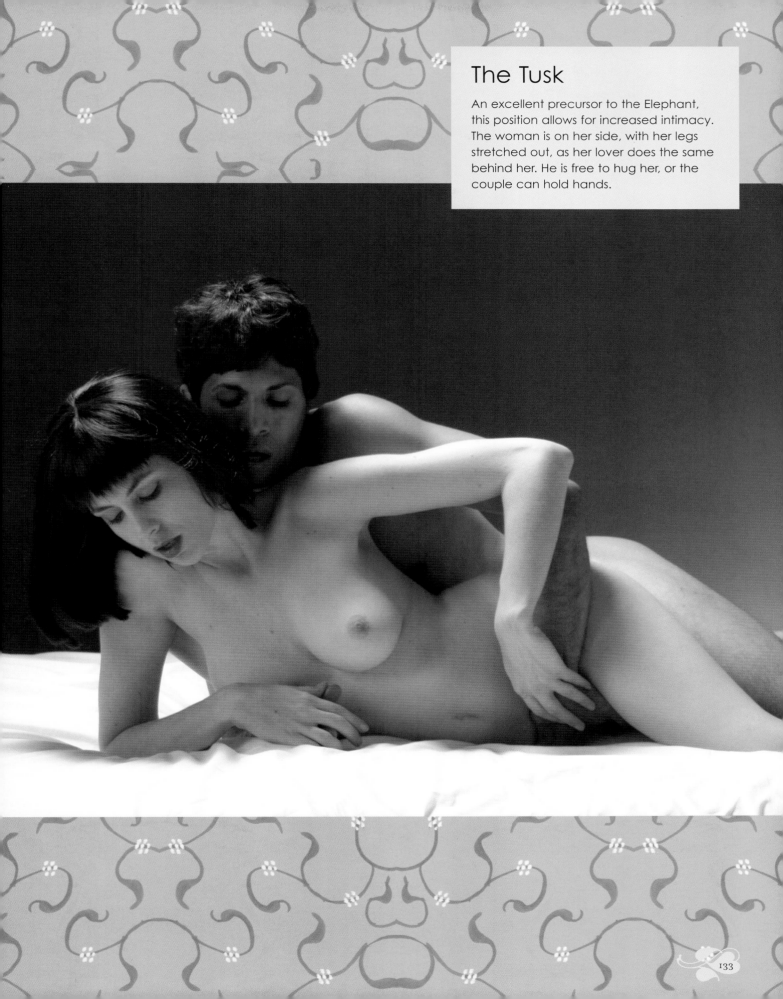

The Tusk

An excellent precursor to the Elephant, this position allows for increased intimacy. The woman is on her side, with her legs stretched out, as her lover does the same behind her. He is free to hug her, or the couple can hold hands.

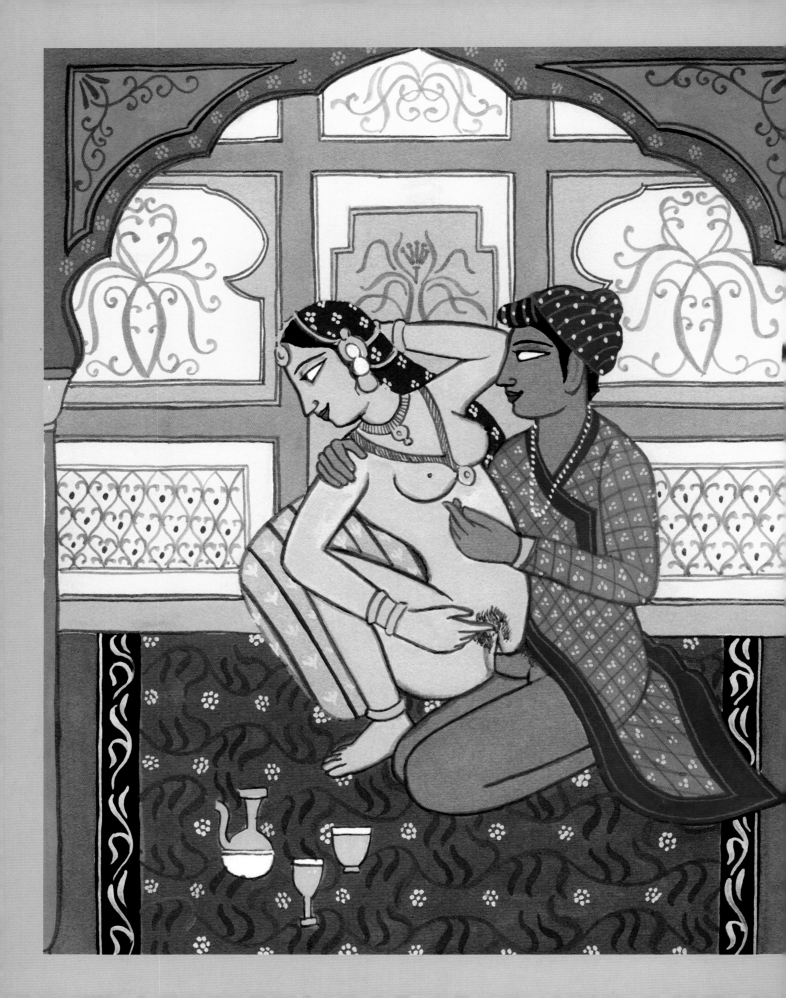

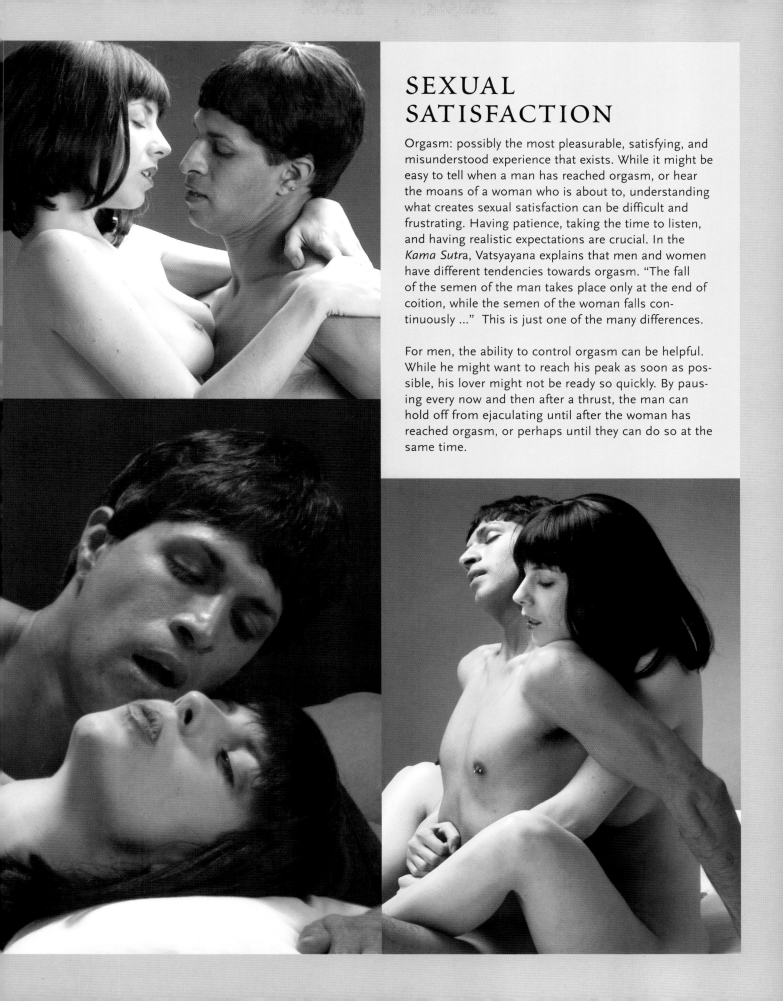

SEXUAL SATISFACTION

Orgasm: possibly the most pleasurable, satisfying, and misunderstood experience that exists. While it might be easy to tell when a man has reached orgasm, or hear the moans of a woman who is about to, understanding what creates sexual satisfaction can be difficult and frustrating. Having patience, taking the time to listen, and having realistic expectations are crucial. In the *Kama Sutra*, Vatsyayana explains that men and women have different tendencies towards orgasm. "The fall of the semen of the man takes place only at the end of coition, while the semen of the woman falls continuously ..." This is just one of the many differences.

For men, the ability to control orgasm can be helpful. While he might want to reach his peak as soon as possible, his lover might not be ready so quickly. By pausing every now and then after a thrust, the man can hold off from ejaculating until after the woman has reached orgasm, or perhaps until they can do so at the same time.

The female orgasm is a bit more complicated. The *Kama Sutra* recognizes the ability for females to have multiple orgasms, and encourages women to fully enjoy the orgasmic experience. For some women, orgasms come easily, for others it is more difficult. By staying in touch with your body, and being creative with your partner, individuals can figure out what works best.

For both the man and woman, it is important to keep an open mind. Not every orgasm will be mind-blowing. Simply focusing on the subtleties of a given moment, like the smell of freshly shampooed hair, the warmth of a naked body pressed against yours, and the soft skin of your partner's neck against your lips, your orgasms will happen naturally. An orgasm shouldn't be the goal of every single love-making session, experimenting with different techniques can increase the likelihood of attaining one.

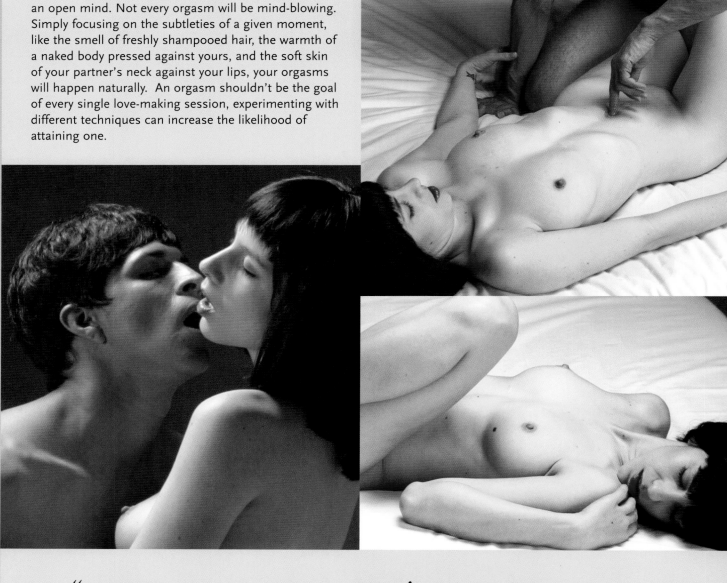

"AN ORGASM SHOULDN'T BE THE GOAL OF EVERY SINGLE LOVE—MAKING SESSION, EXPERIMENTING WITH DIFFERENT TECHNIQUES CAN INCREASE THE LIKELIHOOD OF ATTAINING ONE."

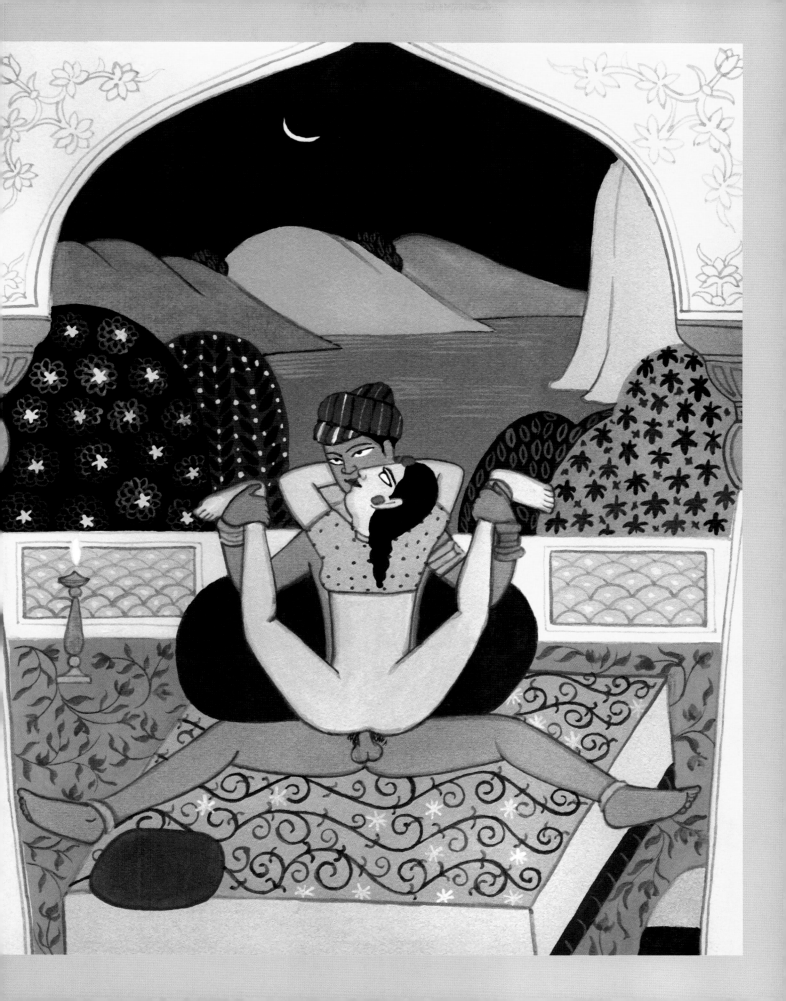

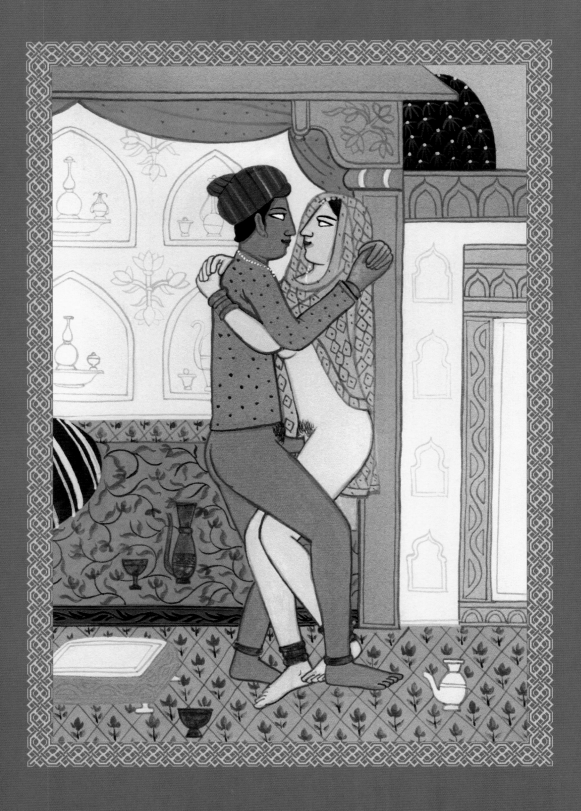

EQUAL POSITIONS

The Equal Positions are meant to increase intimacy and create a feeling of equality. As the couple looks deep into each other's eyes, there will be an openness that occurs, making the partners feel more connected. Often used in tantric sex rituals, these positions will bring the man and woman closer and add new levels of sexual satisfaction.

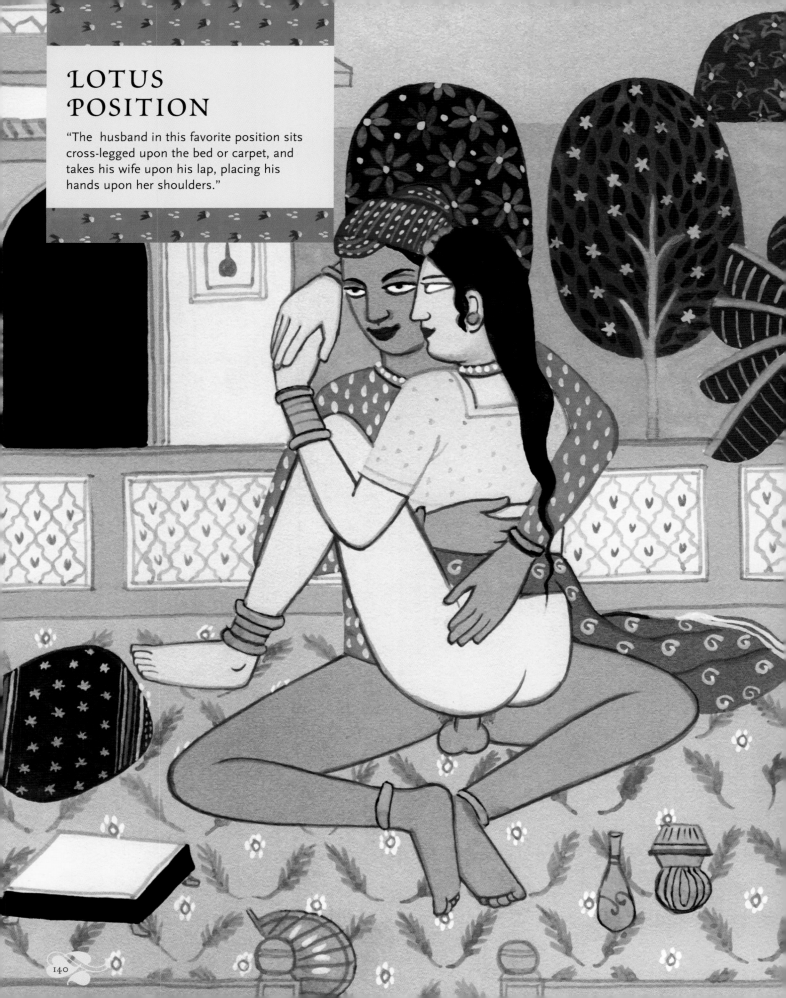

LOTUS POSITION

"The husband in this favorite position sits cross-legged upon the bed or carpet, and takes his wife upon his lap, placing his hands upon her shoulders."

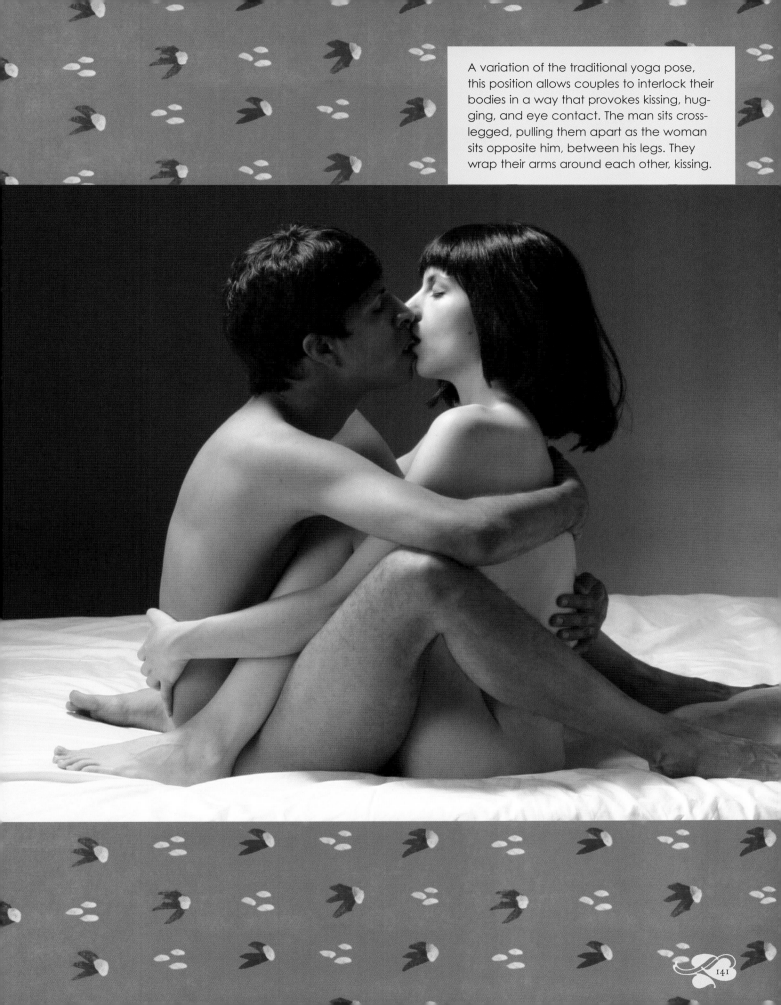

A variation of the traditional yoga pose, this position allows couples to interlock their bodies in a way that provokes kissing, hugging, and eye contact. The man sits cross-legged, pulling them apart as the woman sits opposite him, between his legs. They wrap their arms around each other, kissing.

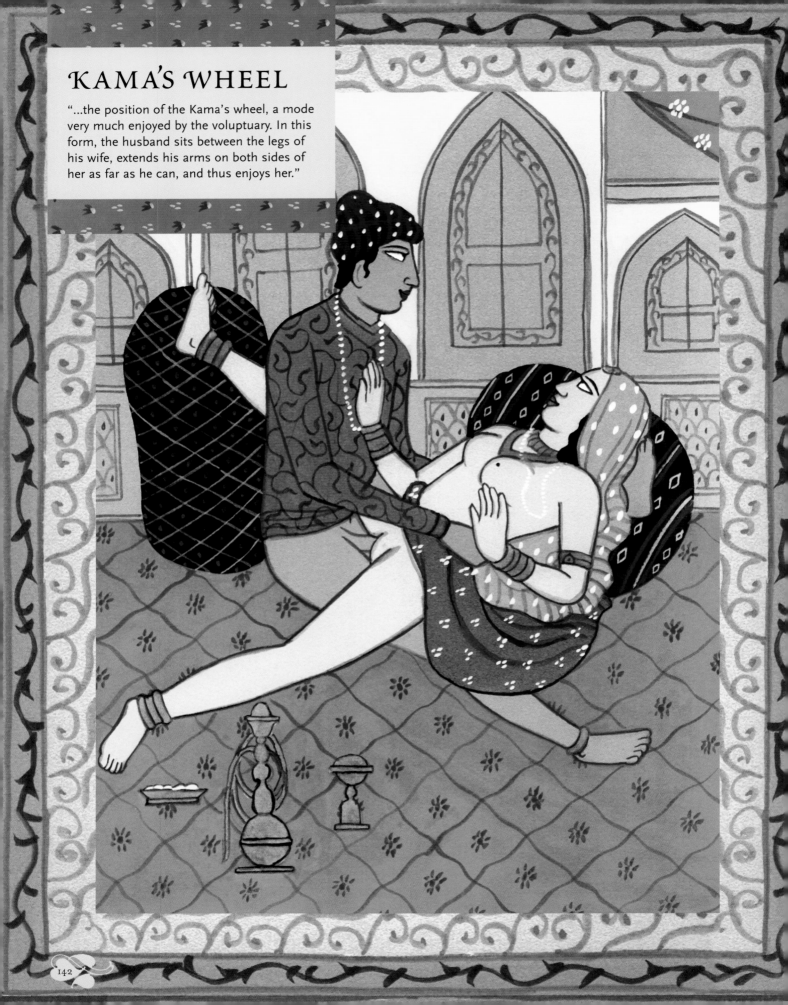

KAMA'S WHEEL

"...the position of the Kama's wheel, a mode very much enjoyed by the voluptuary. In this form, the husband sits between the legs of his wife, extends his arms on both sides of her as far as he can, and thus enjoys her."

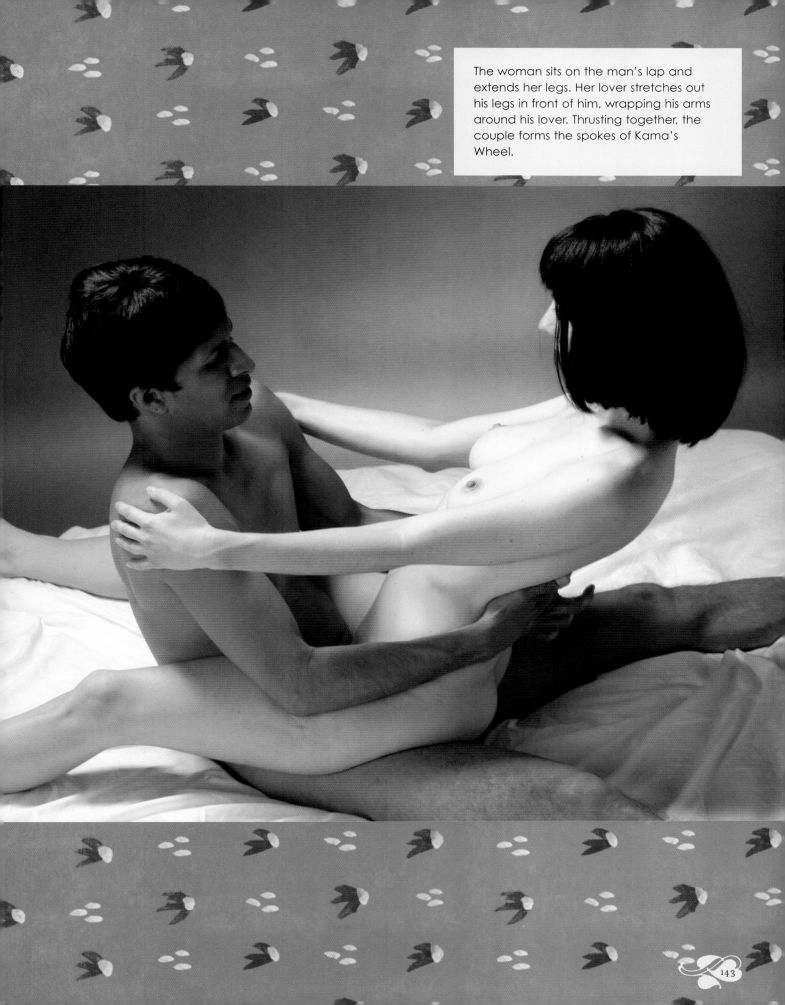

The woman sits on the man's lap and extends her legs. Her lover stretches out his legs in front of him, wrapping his arms around his lover. Thrusting together, the couple forms the spokes of Kama's Wheel.

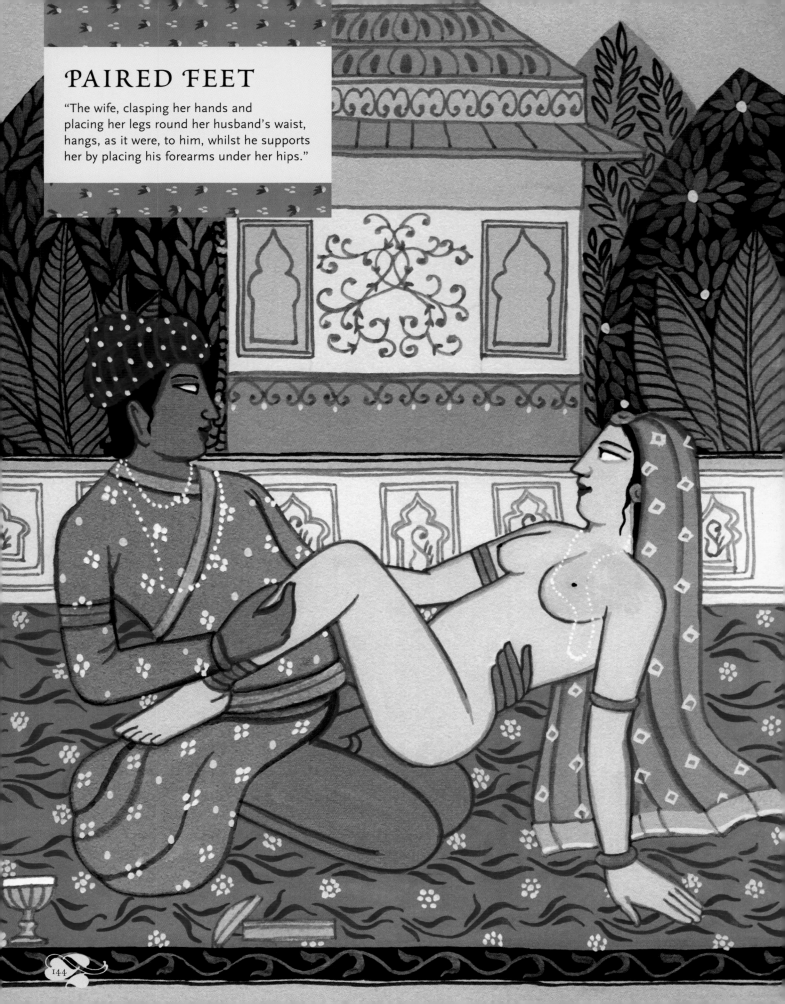

PAIRED FEET

"The wife, clasping her hands and placing her legs round her husband's waist, hangs, as it were, to him, whilst he supports her by placing his forearms under her hips."

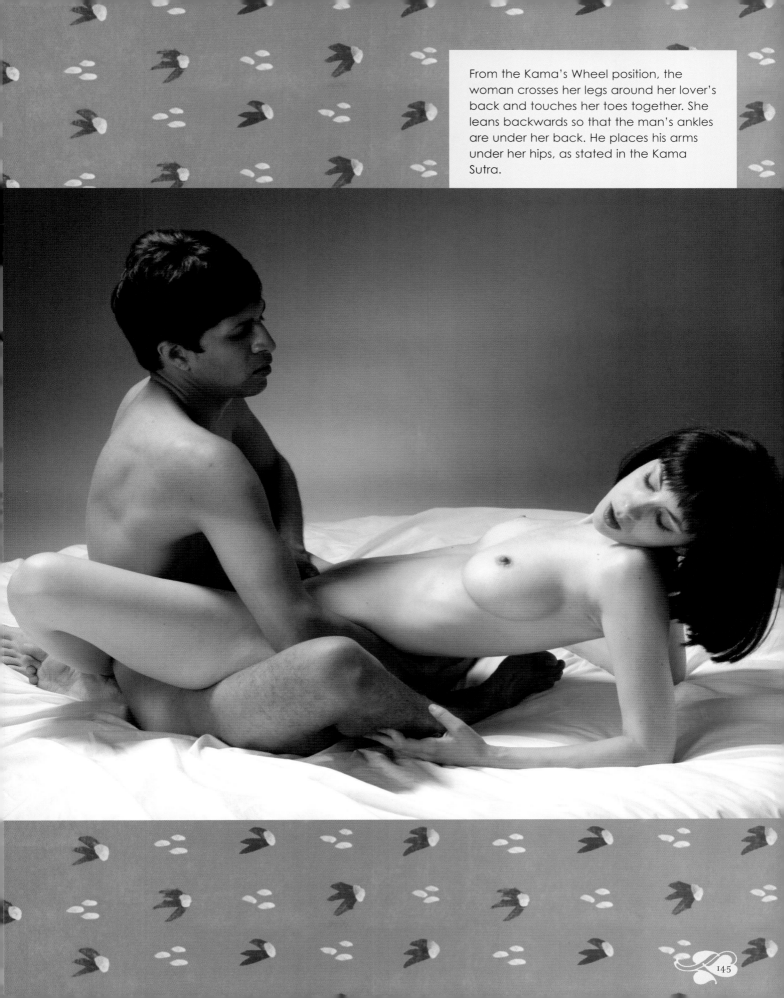

From the Kama's Wheel position, the woman crosses her legs around her lover's back and touches her toes together. She leans backwards so that the man's ankles are under her back. He places his arms under her hips, as stated in the Kama Sutra.

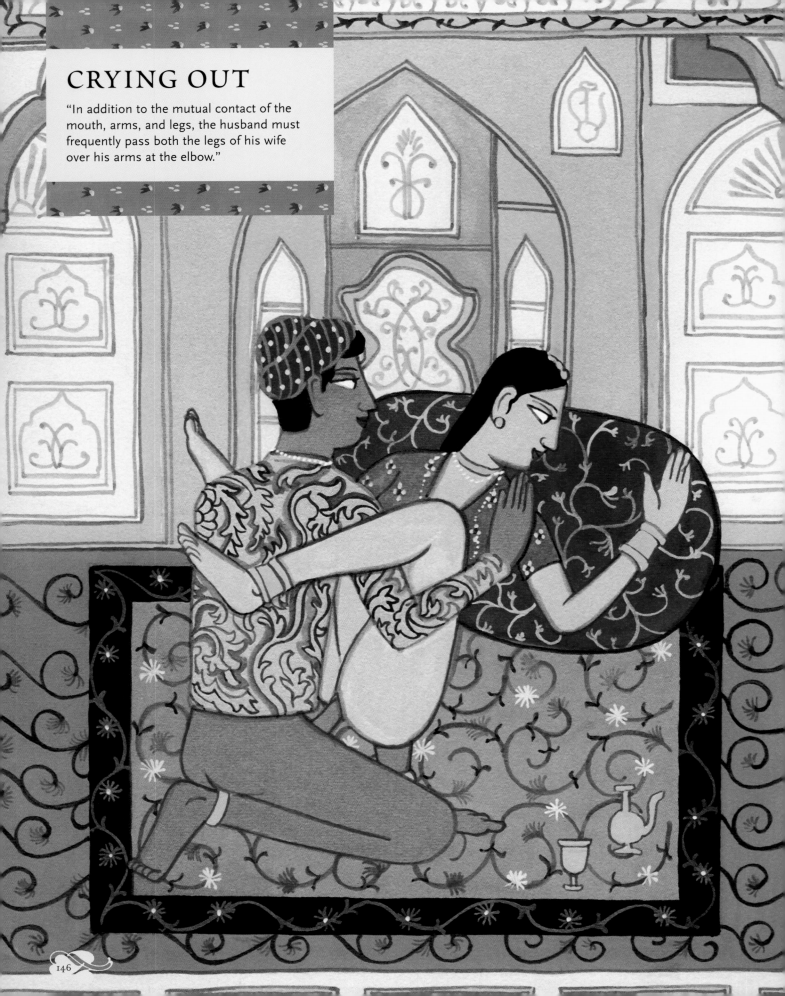

CRYING OUT

"In addition to the mutual contact of the mouth, arms, and legs, the husband must frequently pass both the legs of his wife over his arms at the elbow."

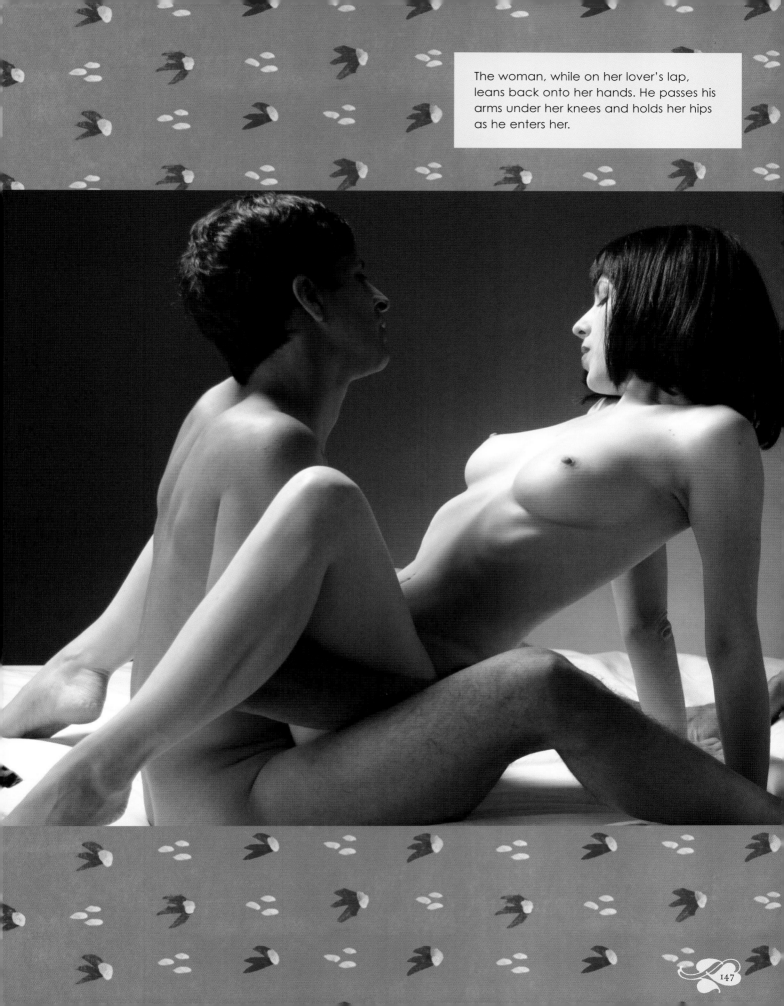

The woman, while on her lover's lap, leans back onto her hands. He passes his arms under her knees and holds her hips as he enters her.

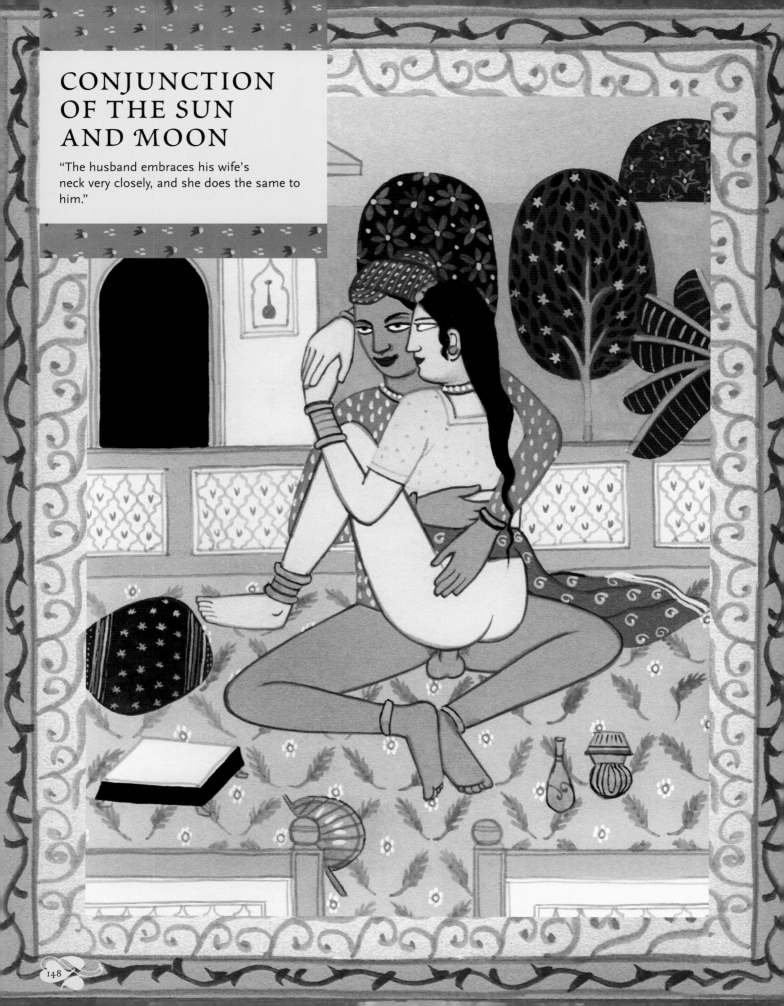

CONJUNCTION OF THE SUN AND MOON

"The husband embraces his wife's neck very closely, and she does the same to him."

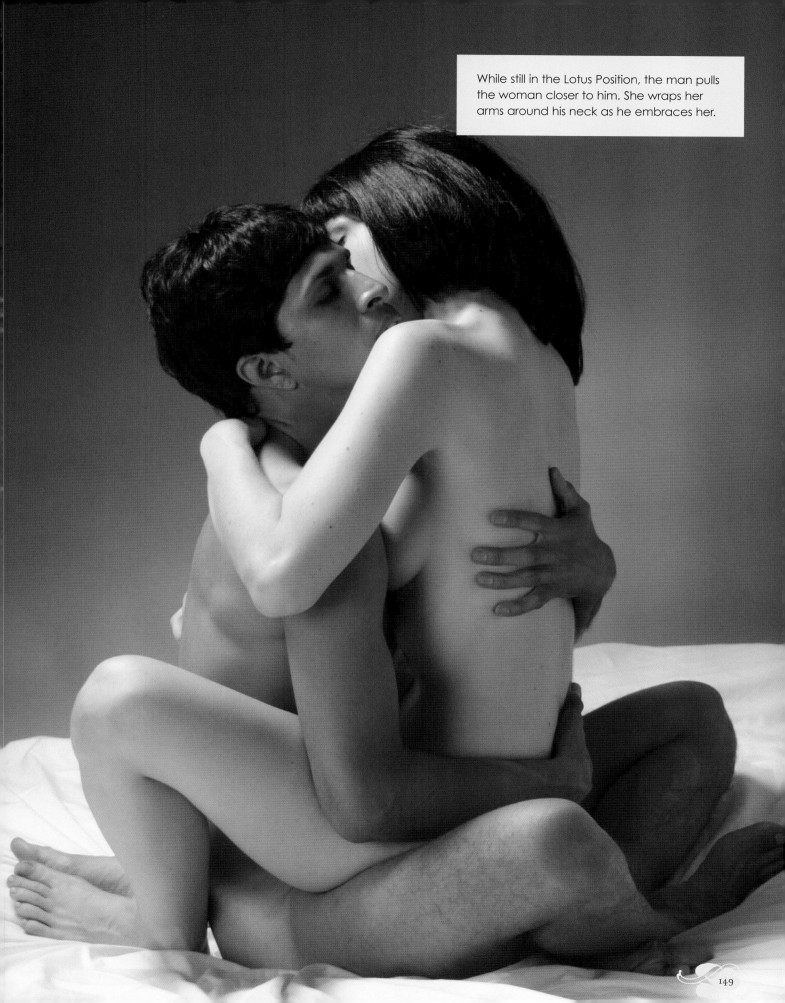

While still in the Lotus Position, the man pulls the woman closer to him. She wraps her arms around his neck as he embraces her.

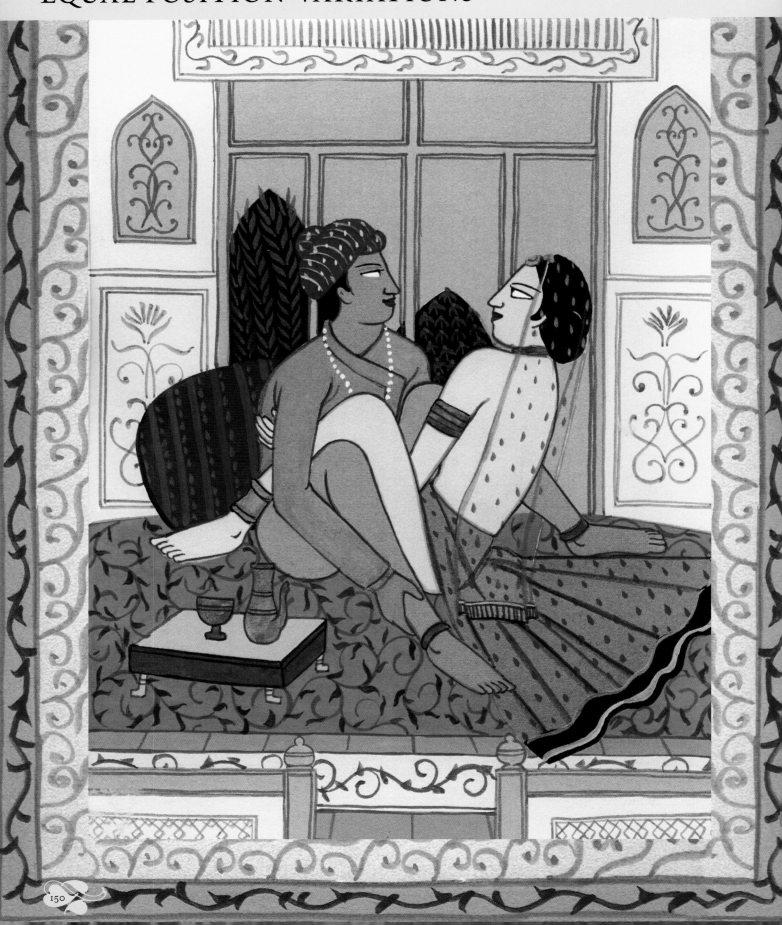

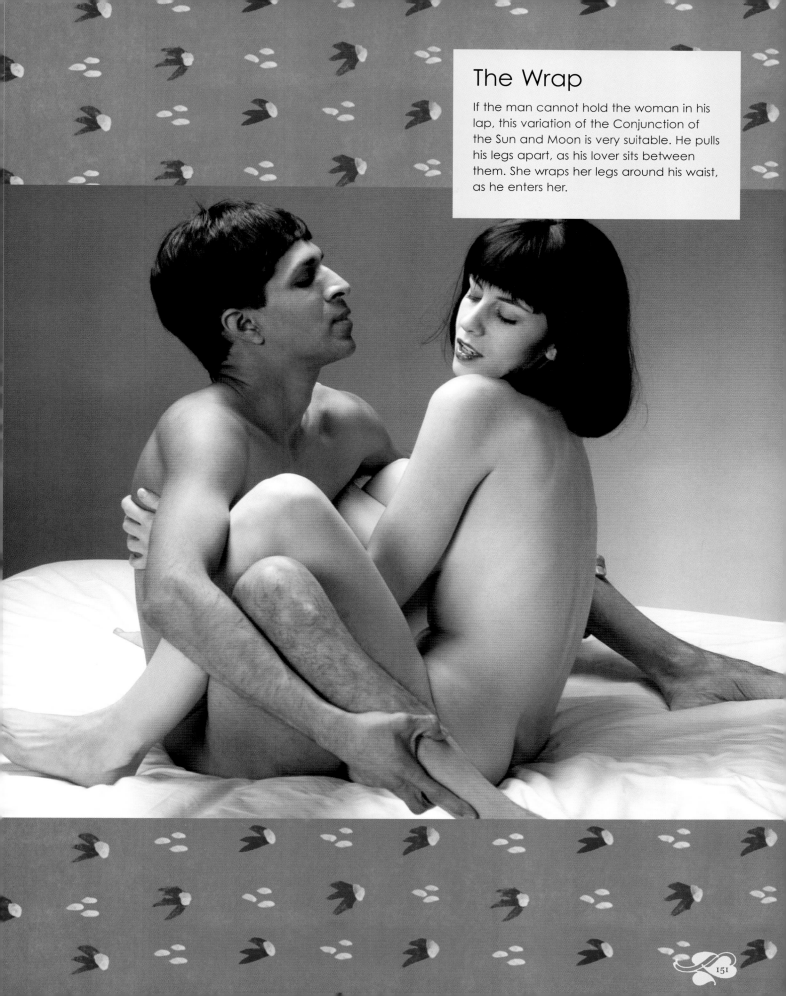

The Wrap

If the man cannot hold the woman in his lap, this variation of the Conjunction of the Sun and Moon is very suitable. He pulls his legs apart, as his lover sits between them. She wraps her legs around his waist, as he enters her.

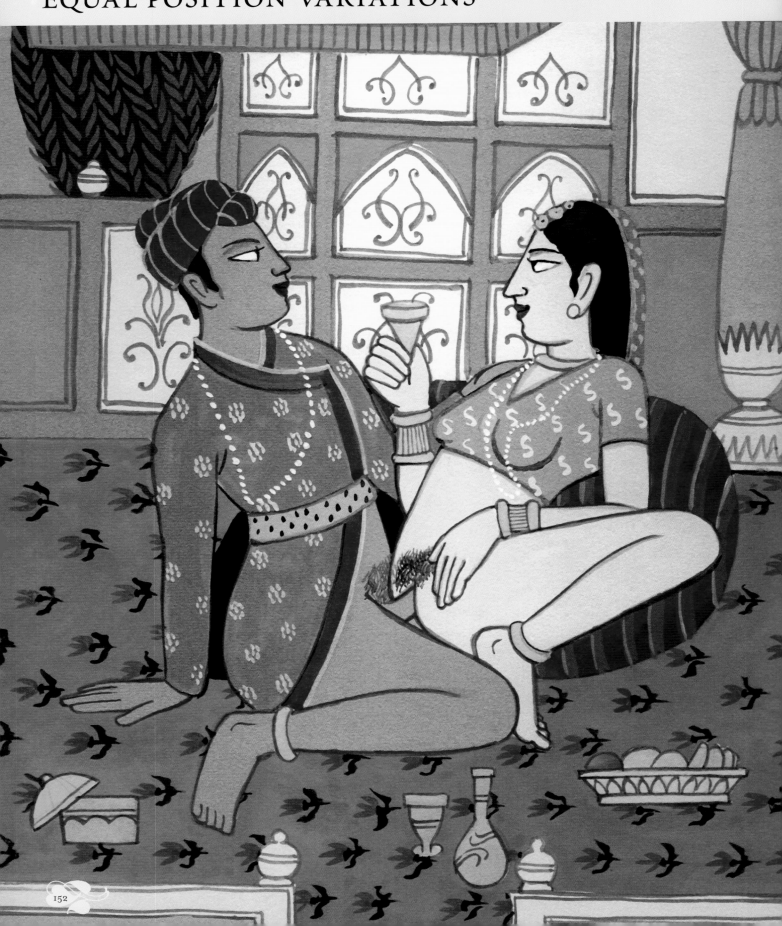

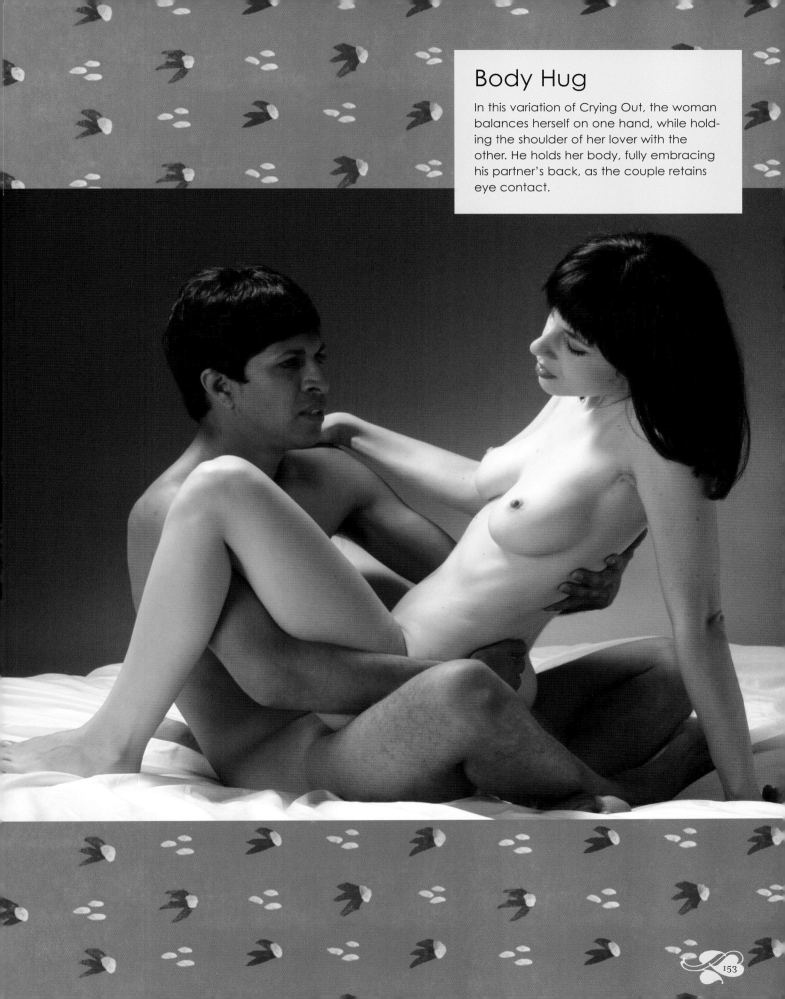

Body Hug

In this variation of Crying Out, the woman balances herself on one hand, while holding the shoulder of her lover with the other. He holds her body, fully embracing his partner's back, as the couple retains eye contact.

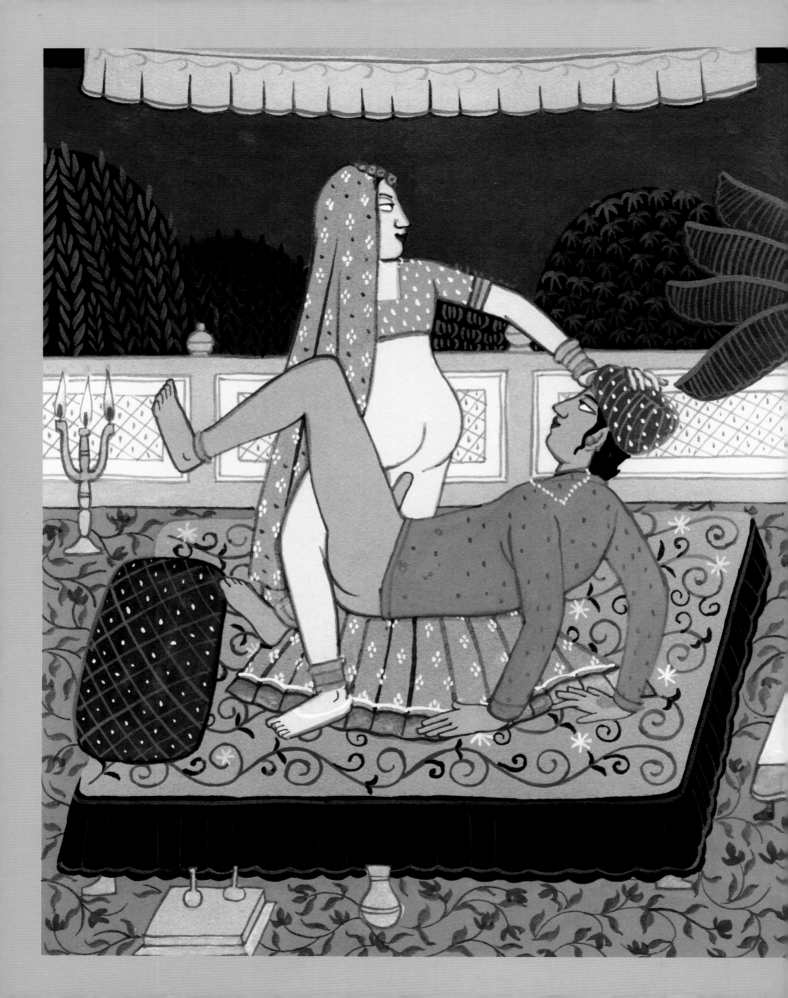

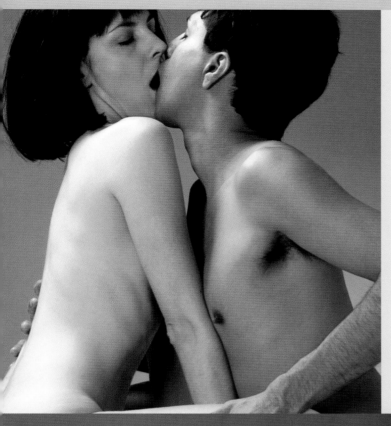

ENHANCING SEXUALITY

Most couples who are looking to enhance their sexual experience start out slowly. The *Kama Sutra* encourages the use of pillows and cushions to help make sex more enticing. The couple can place a pillow under the woman's hips, or the man can kneel on a cushion to make himself more comfortable. Games such as dice were played during the time of Vatsyayana, and by bringing a bit of fun into the bedroom couples will begin to open up to each other.

In the *Kama Sutra*, wide-open spaces were available for engaging in sexual acts. Then, sex was less taboo and not seen as something to be ashamed of. Although Vatsyayana saw congress in water as being prohibited by religious law, he nonetheless recognized that others of the time engaged in it. "... these different ways of lying down, sitting, and standing should be practiced in water, because it is easy to do so therein."

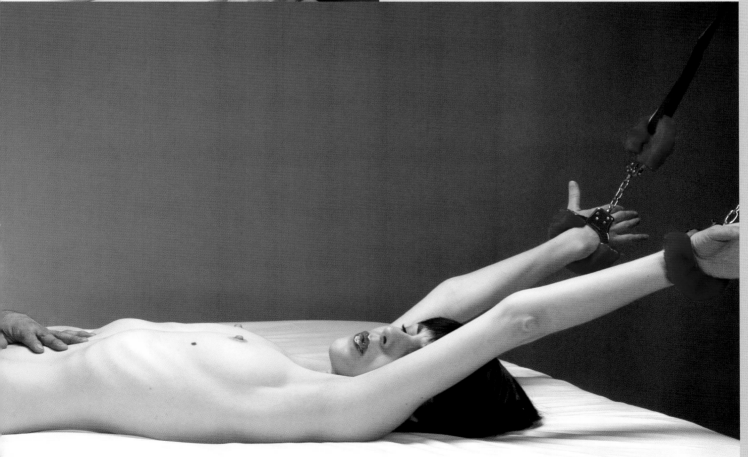

At the time, sex with multiple partners was also accepted. The *Kama Sutra* states, "... many young men enjoy a woman that may be married to one of them, either one after the other, or at the same time." And, "The same things can be done when several men are sitting in company with one courtesan, or when one courtesan is alone with many men. In the same way this can be done by the women of the king's harem when they accidentally get hold of a man." In this way, the couple can, if they feel comfortable, ask others to engage in sex with them. Regardless of what the lovers choose, the two should always remember to make sure it is fun, safe, and enjoyable for whoever is involved.

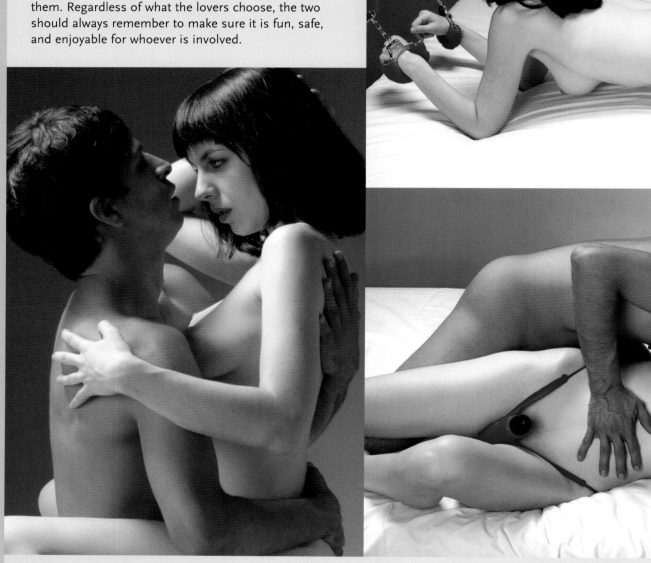

"WITH AN ASSORTMENT OF LUBRICATION PRODUCTS, VIDEOS, AND SEX TOYS OUT THERE, YOU'LL NEVER GET BORED."

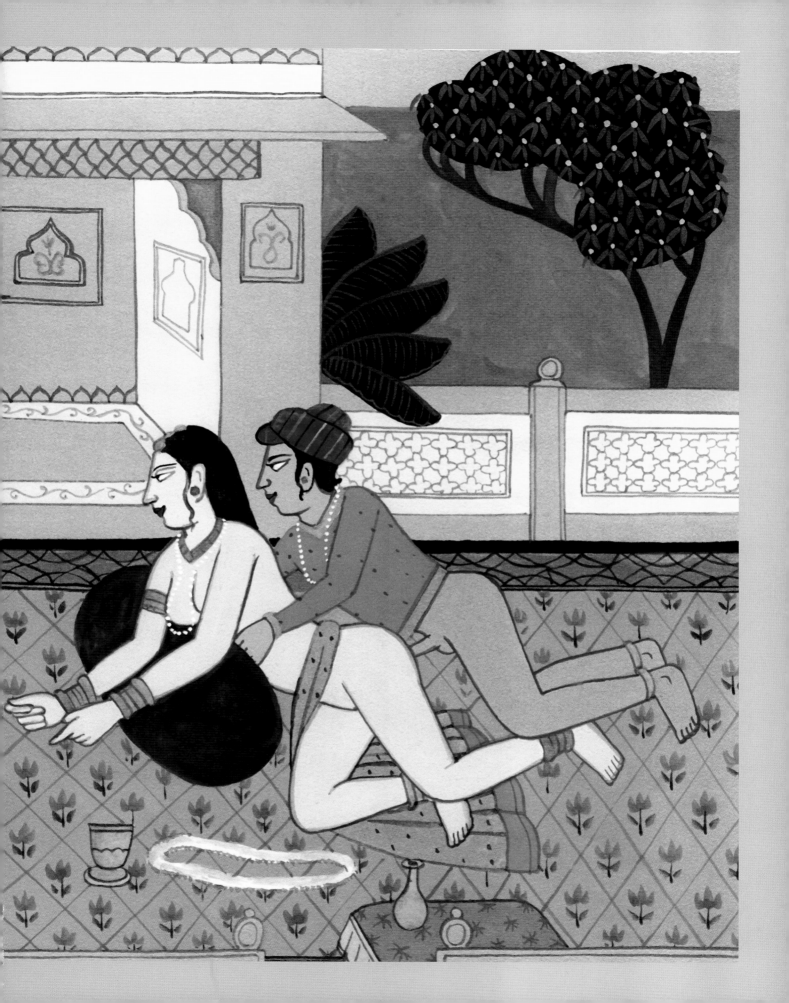

OTHER BOOKS
BY RANDI FOXX:

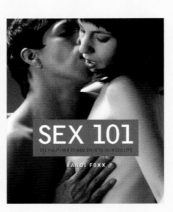

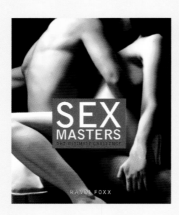

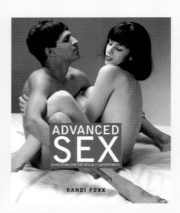

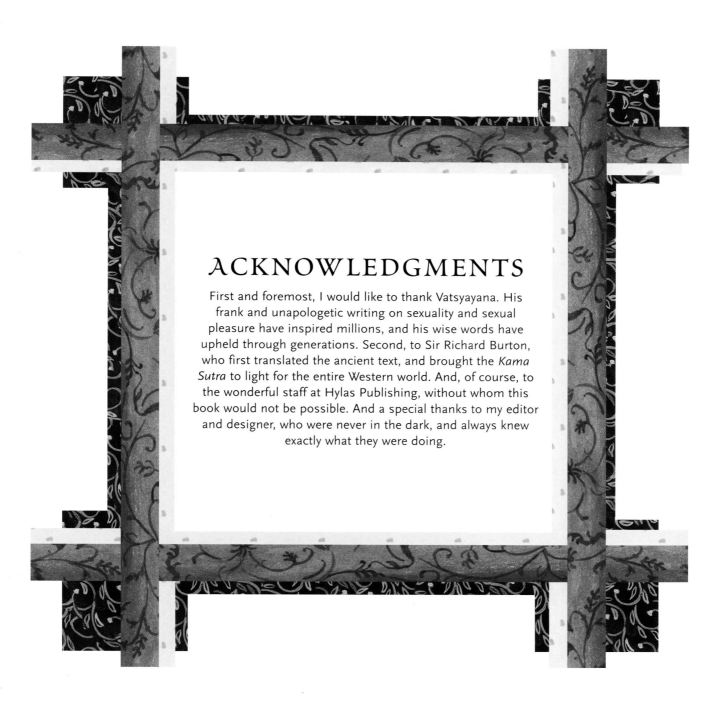

ACKNOWLEDGMENTS

First and foremost, I would like to thank Vatsyayana. His frank and unapologetic writing on sexuality and sexual pleasure have inspired millions, and his wise words have upheld through generations. Second, to Sir Richard Burton, who first translated the ancient text, and brought the *Kama Sutra* to light for the entire Western world. And, of course, to the wonderful staff at Hylas Publishing, without whom this book would not be possible. And a special thanks to my editor and designer, who were never in the dark, and always knew exactly what they were doing.